The Residents' Voice

The Residents' Voice

From a Dementia Unit

Pieta Valentine

To order additional copies of this book, contact:
Xlibris
NZ TFN: 0800 008 756 (Toll Free inside NZ)
NZ Local: 9-801 1905 (+64 9801 1905 from outside New Zealand)
www.Xlibris.co.nz
Orders@Xlibris.co.nz
845847

CONTENTS

Introduction

Daisy, trained as a physiotherapist in 1980s New Zealand when 'ban the bomb', anti-apartheid, and the rise of feminism were fast becoming part of the culture. Physiotherapy school was insular and direct. 'Observe keenly. Collate ample data from the patient, detail all clinical signs, and then make an effective treatment plan for rehabilitation.' This austere approach Daisy dutifully adhered to – lifelong. Modifying though rehabilitation to self-management as she was often left treating the more chronic conditions of geriatrics where rehabilitation wasn't an option.

She was comfortable there, having spent a good part of her childhood as a self-appointed helper, massaging old ladies' knees in her father's medical surgery – with good results and 'Thank you, dear. That's a lot better.'

Daisy worked in various hospitals and clinics overseas before finally settling down in the South Island. After so many years of doing physiotherapy she decided to have a career change and work full time with people who had dementia. She was taken around the dementia unit by the retirement village manager, a mannequin of a woman who must have spent half her night jogging to have kept such a figure. She immediately said Daisy had the job, of diversional therapist, no CV supplied.

She just said, 'It's practically volunteer work here with the wages you'll be getting.'

So be it, thought Daisy. She'd entered the machine, the 24/7 secure dementia unit.

Shut down and shut off from both themselves and each another, it was difficult to know how to help the residents. Daisy tried everything she could think of, but nothing seemed to be working, until Jane, one of the patients, started explaining to her how a person with dementia thinks. Then the residents started responding to an unexpected topic.

Capitalising on this, Daisy coordinated a programme of activities to help them improve their concentration and confidence. Once there, the residents themselves had to take the initiative to communicate independently with one another. After three years, they finally did. From there, they could develop their own community, which they have done – admirably and in a very unique way, making it easier for new residents coming in.

In telling their story and relaying their message, *The Residents' Voice* shares what Daisy learnt from them and offers a unique range of advice and strategies for relatives of dementia patients.

1

Arriving at the Unit

Jane arrived at the unit well dressed in a maroon merino cardigan, a knee-length tan skirt, and cream slingback sandals. After quickly sizing everyone up, she made short work of getting herself sorted. She had the best room, room 1, first on the right and just around the corner from the nurses' station, less likely to get lost and within easy access if she needed help.

She also had the best view. The Southern Alps spread full vista across her window, giving her some much-needed sense of connection with the outside world. A skier in her youth, looking at the mountains somehow realigned her.

Paintings of the family farm adorned her walls, and heavily framed photos of the children's weddings sat on the heavy mahogany chest of drawers. She could count the cars parked outside the bedroom window, noting their vintage, colour, and make any time of the day. Her family didn't know she could still read, so they had not renewed her prescription glasses, but she could make out any number plate, given the chance, within twenty metres. Having to give up driving was one of her most painful memories. She had loved her blue Morris Minor, and it was a sad day when she had to let it go.

And now she had to try to make the most of this cramped situation. There were only the basics in terms of furniture and facilities: a single bed which could be hydraulically raised and lowered, comfortable enough pillows but a bit too spongy for her liking, and crisp white hospital sheets that were too starched to really relax on. At least she still had her favourite mohair blanket. She'd drag it from the bed over to her only half-decent piece of furniture, a comfortable two-seater navy blue corduroy sofa. Deftly set under the window, it neatly caught the afternoon sun. Perfect. Her tiny, five-foot frame fitted into the length of it just right, so she could easily lie down and have an afternoon nap.

Aside from this, there were an overly big chair squashed in the corner at an uncomfortable angle that hardly anyone sat in it, a tapestry footstool that came in handy for putting one's feet on, and a small utilitarian bedside table for her hankies, her lipsticks, her old Girl Guides book, an address book, a diary for appointments, some pens and paper, and various funeral sheets of friends and family sadly gone.

Aside from the adjoining bathroom with the perfunctory toilet, handbasin, and shower, that was it. Oh yes, and the very small wardrobe, behind closed doors, opposite her bed, only enough space for a quarter of the clothes she once had. And her shoes, definitely no space for them, especially the going-out, high-heeled kind. Nevertheless, she had arrived, so she must make the best of it.

Of course, she knew her memory had been fading. But then she'd never had a good memory anyway, which her family had always teased her mercilessly about.

Having surveyed her room for the umpteenth time she decided to poke her head out the door and see what else was around. All she could see was a forbidding long corridor to her right, in which people were walking aimlessly, and on the left the nurses' station, which others in various stages of distress were milling around. Only a portion of the desk was visible. It curved around in a half-U shape so as to serve as part of the walking track leading to the lounge, past the dining room, past the doors of all thirty uniform bedrooms, then back to her own, not unlike a human racecourse.

She noticed over the following weeks that the people on this never-ending walking track seemed to be getting thinner and thinner, whereas the sitting group in the lounge just got fatter and fatter, not their own doing entirely, being fed on such rich cake and biscuits morning, noon, and night. All those people in the lounge – not moving, not talking, not doing anything – she found very sad indeed. Better to stay in her room. She'd never been one to socialise anyway. Life had always been about the farm, the two boys and their rugby, and the two girls with netball and hockey.

She didn't mind her own company most of the time, but she did miss her favourite son, David, whom she hadn't seen yet. She was starting to get distressed about it. She knew he lived up on the farm in North Canterbury, and it was a long drive, but it was still awful not being able to see him. Sometimes uncharacteristically, she'd go to the nurses' station and scream out that she wanted to phone him. But they rarely took any notice, either too busy or not really interested. It was an anguishing time. Having no facility in her room to call and certainly no cell phone, there seemed to be no way of contacting him. She felt like she was pining away. Months seemed to go by like this.

Finally, he arrived. Delighted to see him, she revealed not a bit of her previous anguish. David, tall and handsome with considerable charisma, created quite a stir at the unit. Everyone, it seemed, fell for him. Unperturbed, he set about sorting everything out. He had a real concern for both his mother's and the residents' invisibility and entrapment. The residents loved his company, and he gave willingly and generously of his time in campaigning for them.

He observed how Daisy, the diversional therapist at the unit, had developed a good rapport with his mother. He liked her positive energy and interacting intelligence that was enabling his mother to respond. *That's just what Mum needs*, he thought.

Knowing Daisy was a physio, he asked her if she would see his mother for private treatments. She initially refused, considering it too onerous. But encouraged by David's 'it's for the greater good' persuasion and feeling Jane would be good to work with, she accepted. Appointments were set for every Monday morning.

Jane, by now, was well used to lying on her bed for most of the day and in no way liked to be disturbed. Daisy arriving was an intrusion. She would challenge her with 'What are we doing all this for?' When Daisy explained it was at David's initiation, that would generally appease her.

They started with outside walks, putting on decent walking shoes in the summer, and making sure to wrap up warmly in the winter. Initially, Jane was not keen; but persevering, they eventually found some common ground.

The first discovery was that Jane enjoyed meeting, greeting, and waving to the confined residents over at the hospital wing. She liked the from-a-distance socialising – a big win. Communicating one on one, though, proved to be more difficult. After being challenged with 'I don't mind being made to walk, but I dislike being made to talk', it took a lot of creativity on Daisy's part to get any sort of communication going.

Daisy started to notice Jane liked the large scenic pictures lining the hospital corridors, especially those featuring lakes, rivers, and rowing boats. So they started to slow down and talk about these as they walked by. Jane said her father had bad knees, so they both used to row along the river through the farm to save him from having to walk.

Near these paintings of boats, there was a large world map with New Zealand placed way at the bottom. One day Daisy remarked to Jane how close New Zealand was to the Antarctic, literally at the bottom of the world, to which Jane gave the considered reply, 'Good to see we are still functioning.'

From what little Jane said, it was obvious she was astute, but it was difficult to get to know her much more. Often after just a one-liner, she'd typically clam up, saying, 'I don't want to talk all the time.' If she was in a receptive mood, Daisy would be lucky to get two lines out of her but rarely more. It went on like this for months.

When Jane didn't want to get up for their Monday morning walk, she'd just curl right up, refusing to budge. Most of the time, though, she obliged; and once outside, she enjoyed both the walk and the socialising. Over the months, connection had built, so Daisy thought it time to push for more information.

She'd never had the chance to work privately with a dementia patient as she was doing with Jane. When working as a physiotherapist in hospital settings, she'd be lucky to get twenty minutes with anyone, thirty minutes max, and then only for a limited number of treatments. Here with Jane, she had a full hour – often extended into personal time so as to get that little bit more.

She'd become interested in the psychology of the dementia experience mainly because she wanted to be able to help these people. She couldn't see whether she would be able to do that if she didn't understand what they were thinking and experiencing. She was keen to find out more and had the inkling Jane would be the one to explain it to her. She decided to pursue this at the next available opportunity.

Daisy knew Jane disliked answering questions. She'd made that clear, especially when withdrawn into her defiant comatose position, code for *Get out and leave me alone*. It was going to be a fine balancing act.

After spending the extra time with Jane, a friendship was developing. Occasionally, after work, Daisy would come to Jane's room and sit and watch the sun disappear over the Alps. They were special moments. A magical calm seemed to descend when that crimson sunset pink, backed by the last sky blue, disappeared over the back of the peaks. Jane went to sleep happily after that, with Daisy a little calmer after what was often a hectic day at work.

Walking into Jane's room the next Monday morning, Daisy found her retracted, so she expected the angry 'Get away!' This time, she didn't get it. Jane just lay there, refusing to move, her thin frame curled up, facing the wall resolutely.

Daisy felt the timing was right. She had a hunch she might get something from her.

It was mid-May but a nice day, not too cold. By eleven, it had warmed up a bit, so now was a good time to get outside – if Jane was prepared to get off her bed. Daisy started with the usual preliminaries. 'Good morning, Jane. It's Monday morning, the day for our walk. It's a lovely day out there, so it would be good to get out. We can have a walk, then sit at our favourite seat by the rose garden.'

Daisy didn't expect her to get up – she rarely did when in this state – but she hoped she could extend the olive branch enough to soften her into saying something. Jane refused to answer.

'Come on, Jane. Let's make use of the day. It's beautiful out there.'

Again, a stony silence.

Daisy abruptly changed tack. 'Why not? Why don't you want to get up?'

No response.

More assertively now, 'Why not get up and come out?'

Instead of going back as usual to the blue sofa to wait, Daisy stood her ground. Raising herself to her full height, she just stood there, waiting. *As long as it takes.*

'Why not?'

'Why not, Jane?'

'Tell me.'

Finally relenting, Jane said quietly, 'Fuzzy brain.'

Able to soften her stance, Daisy said, 'Thank you, Jane. I really appreciate that.' *At last, the first glimpse, a clue.* It felt like the first find on an archaeological dig.

Three weeks later, Daisy had some more. She disliked agitating Jane when in her self-induced comatose state, but that was precisely the time she could get the answers she needed. Being assertive was the only way to get them. Pleasant and persuasive never elicited anything. So the next time Jane was curled up and reclusive, Daisy persevered, asking, Why do you get a fuzzy brain?'

After several stony silences, Jane spat out, 'Fuzzy mind.'

'Do you mean a racing mind?' Daisy asked.

'Yes!'

'Thank you, Jane. That's a great help. No more questions.'

One question a week was more than enough. Daisy knew Jane hated all this prying. This made for slow progress, but Daisy was happy having all she needed to get started. A racing mind is essentially a stressed-out mind. From here, she could start to make some headway.

She was beginning to feel mildly optimistic. She always felt it was never going to be some medical-type miracle or a vaccine approach. Dementia was psychological, not physical, after all and just the memory part of the psyche involved. Psychology was Daisy's interest as she'd been a life long meditator and read a lot about it. She loved the depth and detail. On top of that, forty years as a physio had filled her with a down-to-earth pragmatism. Though she liked the theory of psychology, she needed to see it translated to practical benefit; otherwise, she couldn't see the point and generally wouldn't rest until she had.

They now needed a topic to work with. Daisy asked Jane what she'd like to work on, and without hesitation, she said clear as a bell, 'Confidence.' No hesitation there. Jane explained that her confidence had plummeted with the memory loss. Being beholden pained her, having to rely so much on others.

Daisy had to think about what methodology to use to rebuild Jane's confidence. Pooling together all sources, she discovered Jane liked anything to do with motivation, mental strength, discipline, and positive thinking, much of it harking back to her sporting days. This was quite an arsenal to work with, and Daisy could see Jane was ready to work with it all.

The first Monday was 'Think strong. Be strong.' They discussed all aspects. What does it mean to be strong? How to develop mental strength? What type of attitude do you need? What experiences help? What strong character inspires?

After the lesson, Daisy wrote it up with thick black felt-tip pen in big large letters on a good-sized card and placed it on Jane's small bedside table, angled towards her for her to best see when lying down. 'Think strong. Be strong.' Jane would lie on her bed and look at it at length, thinking about it. Sometimes Daisy would see her carrying it around the corridor with her in the same way others transported their treasured dolls.

With each lesson, Jane liked to have her new mind-training card by her bed at all times, so she could 'look at it and think about it' and 'keep it front of my mind.'

'I like to think about it, the good thinking,' she'd say. And Daisy could see she actually was thinking.

Daisy did one lesson on mental discipline. She got out her laptop and brought up the eight-minute video of Torvill and Dean's 1984 Olympic-winning 'Bolero' routine. Jane was transported.

In time, though, Daisy realised it was more the theoretical, esoteric discussion that Jane preferred, less cluttered and easier to apply to her own thinking. Daisy had always enjoyed such topics, so there was no shortage of material to go on.

Good thinking, positive thinking, was Jane's favourite. So many variations. What was good thinking? What is a good attitude? A good life? Good relationships? Good aims? Good approach? You name it, Daisy and Jane discussed it.

Not just the topic but two or three motivational quotes were also now written up on the card, so Jane had more to think about over the week. The card from the fifth of December 2018 said:

Intelligence is the most important.
Use it by thinking, understanding, and enjoying.
Don't worry about the memory and mind.

To this, Jane said, 'I need to keep that going, nice things. I use a lot of those things. I try to think nice things. Don't you?' Confidence was building, and trust was building further.

Jane could see Daisy was putting in the time and the effort. She was reliable and never missed a Monday.

Still, there were flare-ups, generally triggered by 'They don't understand.' At such times, Jane was loud and overly assertive. 'Get out. I don't want you here. I said out!' For someone who otherwise didn't want to talk very much, at times like this, she was loud. When triggered and after the outburst, Jane wasn't interested in anything – not walking, not talking, not listening. Nothing would console her. Nothing reassured.

There was only one thing that worked, and that was phoning David. He had a remarkable ability to de-escalate her. His rich, mellow voice worked wonders.

Also, he was the only one in the family who'd take the time, especially since Jane had come to the unit, to really understand her, appreciate her efforts, and, if need be, sort out problems if they arose. Her other children, when visiting, had their own views of what was happening and were not really interested in her world as it was now. They had fixed ideas of how things should be, so they couldn't see it from her point of view. They thought all that was important was that she was cared for properly.

Jane was enjoying the intellectual stimulation of the sessions, which she called 'the Thinking Training', sometimes saying they were 'Mind Training'. She said, 'They're good for my confidence.' Thinking had always been important to Jane. She'd learnt to rely on it all her life, compensating for a poor memory. It was good to get back to it again.

Jane's life had always been busy, with everything about being purposeful and constructive. She knew most of the women in the unit were happy sitting with one another in the lounge, often dozing off while watching television. She'd never do that, she said. She didn't like seeing the women just sitting there, not moving, not saying anything. She didn't like just sitting around.

There had never been time for that in her life, and even if there had been, she wasn't interested. No time. There were always the kids and all their sport and then the weeds and tussocks that always needed to be sprayed and pulled out on the farm.

All her life, she told Daisy, it was really only David who had ever understood her or had an interest in what was important. That was why they had such an affinity.

She'd accumulated her stack of thinking cards keenly, and in no time, her top drawer was bulging. She rotated them as fast as her neighbours did their teddy bears. She loved the sessions with Daisy, she said. Monday was now her favourite day. 'This is me learning. It's good for my brain.'

Each week was spent getting a worthy enough quote and card to put beside her bed, quite an undertaking for Daisy, especially when Jane was in little mood for talking. There was a conflict between her 'I don't want to talk all the time' and 'I like to have a card I can think about.' After all, Daisy had to know what Jane wanted written on the card! Each week, though, a card of some sort managed to be propped up in its rightful place.

Not concerned with the writing style (Daisy's printing was scrawly due to an old hand injury), Jane thought the cards 'just lovely'. Sometimes Daisy drew a little boat with a setting sun to give it artistic flair. Staff must have wondered what all these cards were about, but as Jane clearly liked them, they generally left them where they were. To the credit of her main carer, Angela, who was very good to Jane, most of them stayed.

Meanwhile, sometimes walking and always talking continued to be a considerable effort for Jane. There was one helpful skill she didn't resist, though – eye contact. That was easy and natural for her. It was more subtle and less gross than having to force herself to speak. She would cooperate with that any time. It proved to be extremely helpful for Jane as her speech was a lot more fluent when she could hold Daisy's gaze. She would trail off quickly without it. Eye contact was also helpful for Daisy as she could more easily gauge where Jane was at in terms of mood and emotion.

Her attention and concentration were vastly improved with this practice, and no matter what her mood, she welcomed the 'look in the eyes' reminders. 'It's good for me,' she said.

2

Over-Medication

Just as Jane was starting to make good progress, an ominous letter arrived. It was addressed to Jane's Power of Attorney (POA) stating Jane was 'aggressive to staff and attacking residents without reason'. It was signed by the clinical manager.

This spelt doom for both Jane and Daisy's work with her. Daisy knew there was no justification for the accusation, which was based on an attack that another dementia resident who disliked Jane said happened, but there was no other witness and no evidence notes. It seemed incredible to Daisy that such a letter was even written.

David was flabbergasted. Something about it didn't ring true, he thought. He started to think back to previous comments carers had made to him about Jane and started making his own investigations. Angela told him, 'I haven't seen aggression in Jane.'

The weekend carer said, 'Jane is good now at getting to her room. She has been happy for months and fine when helping her with showering and dressing.'

Consoled by these comments, David set about getting Jane's records to see what was written in them. By now, he knew aggression and attacks had to be recorded to be quoted. He was told that to get the notes, he had to go through Jane's POA. This was his elder sister, so he couldn't see there would be a problem, but when he asked for them, she put up strong resistance.

David eventually retrieved them but only after an exhausting round of complex negotiations, going back and forth to the charge nurse and whoever else was on duty and had clout at the time. As he'd expected, there was no documentation of either aggression to staff or attacking another resident. So there was no incriminating evidence, but it was still all hell's job to turn the tide.

Having done his homework, David knew that if Jane was sent to a higher-level dementia care unit (which was what the letter was insinuating), her quality of life would quickly drop. If not that, then the charge of aggression meant that heavy medication would be prescribed, and you didn't have to look very far around the unit to see the results of that clearly on display. Easy to do when relatives are neither questioning or challenging.

At the next level up, residents lay in lines outside the unit in pram-like chairs – outside because they'd never escape. Many hadn't stood up for years. The ones inside the unit were mobile but often violent, so they'd get restrained. It gave a psychiatric ward feel to it – maybe not for the carers working there but certainly for uninitiated visitors.

Then of course, Jane would lose her view, her treasured link to the outside world. Few rooms in such places had a view worth noting and certainly not her Alpine panorama. Spurred on by this knowledge, David threw himself into the minefield, which it most certainly was. He had to correspond at length with the village manager, village clinical manager, unit clinical manager, and charge nurse to get through all the bureaucratic and logistical maze. It seemed it was all set up to either confuse or derail. Having not been challenged on such matters before, the medical establishment's hackles were raised and blood pressures ran high. Unperturbed, David waded through it all, stated his case, asked the right questions, met the right people, spoke at the necessary family meetings, doctors' meetings, and clinical meetings, and eventually turned the tables.

Jane was able to stay at the unit. It was a herculean effort, the first turnaround of its kind. David had broken the back of it.

From then on, access to residents' notes was made easier, and relatives more readily asked for them. More conscientious verbal updates were now given by staff to relatives rather than the previous pious platitudes of 'Your mother's just a little bit agitated so needs more medication.' Such an innocuous but lethal statement and especially seemingly benign when it came from a cherub-faced Filipino nurse.

David hadn't been quick enough though. Jane had already been medicated up. The doctor had already been informed by the unit clinical manager of the so-called attacks and had charted the increase. The side effects of this over-medication were colossal. Jane developed Parkinson's-type symptoms. Jane's previously long strong strides were now replaced by unstable shuffling steps, which were getting faster and faster in pace and smaller and smaller in stride length, so eventually, she'd get tripped up.

Daisy would often find Jane walking along the corridor at an accelerating speed, distressed and breathless, trying to find her room. She explained to Jane how to take longer steps to override the shuffle, but Jane often forgot so had multiple falls as a result. Jane had better balance reactions than most from all the work on the farm and her sporting days, but still, the falls were hard and a terrible blow to her confidence.

David worked with the doctor, feeding back to him Jane's symptoms so he could better adjust the medication, a tricky process as Jane was now getting a restless rigidity in her whole body and couldn't even relax on lying down, so she had lost her once secure haven. The restlessness made her want to lie down and then sit up in quick succession, often every couple of minutes. It was exhausting for Jane and anyone else witnessing it. No amount of persuasion or relaxation therapy could settle it. Her symptoms reduced only when the medication doses were finally stabilised.

Stable medication helped reduce the rigidity, but a safe walking pattern still needed to be retrained and regained and direction orientation improved so she could once again find her room. Fortunately, Daisy's physiotherapy training helped with that, but Jane's confidence had been knocked to the core. She'd always relied on her fast, smart walking pace to bolster her. To be without it now was a massive blow. Finding her room had always been difficult, but generally, sometimes with a bit of direction assistance from a carer, she'd get there. Now she was finding it next to impossible, even when staff gave her directions and even though it was the easiest room to get to, first on the right after the nurses' station.

She was now vulnerable to scathing comments. Worse still, it was totally exhausting. Having to go round and round that never-ending corridor track until some able person, usually a carer or relative, guided her back was dispiriting. She'd ask many a wandering resident, but they rarely knew the way to her room. Most were finding it hard enough to get back to their own. It was difficult to know whom to ask, especially when the 'racing mind and fuzzy brain' kicked in. Disorientated, she was at everyone's mercy.

After a particularly bad spell, Daisy finally came to see her and asked how she was. Jane said, 'I can feel myself slipping.'

'How so?'

'I don't feel right. I'm doing my best, but it is hard.'

'And you are walking?'

'Not that wonderful, but I'm getting from A to B.'

So they started the training sessions with just that, getting from A to B. The start A was at the big red metal roses hanging on the wall opposite the nurses' station, the official start, from there to Jane's room. Typical instructions were, 'Stride out, Jane, big steps. Keep going. Lift your feet . . . through the doors. Look to your right, first on the right. Look for the sign. Look for your name. Look for your room number. No, that's the wrong way. You've overstepped. Back up now. Now look again for your name, your room.' Then eventually, 'Good. Well done, Jane. You've found it, your room. You're here. Congratulations.'

'Thank god for that,' Jane would say.

'You're doing really well. I can see you're working hard.'

'I'm trying hard. No point in doing it otherwise.'

Jane never tired of it. She was heroic – back and forth, forth and back. Slowly but surely, she was getting there.

David would practise the same routine with her when he came to visit as would, to a lesser extent, the rest of the family. The biggest help, though, came when the carers and nurses started to chime in, 'Room 1, first on the right, Jane, first on the right.' This repetitive room reminder affirmation helped a lot.

Daisy stuck yet another laminated card (someone was taking them) on her door with Blu-Tack, lower down and in bigger letters so Jane could see it more clearly. She was short, and the standard high-up sign was difficult to see. So there now at Jane's eye level was, 'Jane's room. Room 1.'

The hundreds of practice runs were starting to sink in. Her gait was improving, her steps getting longer, her strides getting stronger. It all seemed to be slowly starting to work.

Yet still, Jane was having a hard time of it. Everything seemed to hang in the balance. Any small thing could tip her. There were so many things that didn't seem right and weren't going well. And there seemed to be so few people to ask and get help from with the ever-mounting problems. Unbeknown to others, Jane's feet were getting worse. She was having increasing difficulty walking on them.

When Daisy next visited, Jane said on standing, 'My toe hurts.'

Daisy took off Jane's shoes, and there was a great, big inflamed red bunion on her right toe. *Oh no. That's going to cause problems.*

She'd been having twice weekly shiatsu foot massages ever since she'd come in, Daisy knew, so why hadn't the beautician masseuse doing the treatments picked up the problem? She was treating the feet, so surely, she couldn't have missed it. *It will take an age to get to the chiropodist. And who will make all the enquiries?* Daisy knew it would be her.

It took eight requests over the next three weeks to various people in the chain of command to make sure the chiropodist was indeed coming in and, yes, would be coming regularly, and Jane's name would be put in the diary, and yes, it was all in place and sorted. *Whew.*

Next, the shoes had to be worked out. It was pretty obvious the glamorous cream sling-backs were no longer going to work nor the pinching-the-toe patent leather kind or any of the others for that matter. All were too tight and gave no room for the bunion. In the end, there was only one pair of battered brown Hush Puppies that fitted, giving just enough room so the bunion would not be compressed.

Making enquiries to the family to get another pair of shoes seemed to need a lot of justifying and explaining. 'Are they really needed?'

Well, yes. What if this last Hush Puppies pair got lost? Worn out? Ruined? What with summer coming up?

What about taking Jane to a specialist shoe shop that knows about bunion fitting? Yes, they can be expensive. But what about looking out for the sales? It would help Jane enormously in her walking ability if she could just get one more decent pair of shoes. So a cascade of refundable unsuitable shoes arrived. Sporty-looking a lot of them, too tight and not right.

So in the end, with the Hush Puppies long gone, Jane resorted to a pair of too big, too floppy blue velvet slippers.

This must have been demoralising too. It was substandard, whichever way you looked at it.

The training – and support required for that – now seemed to be covering an ever-expanding portfolio for Daisy. But she battled on nevertheless.

Cold weather was now creeping in, so that needed to be dealt with. She bustled around, trying to find Jane's winter set of woollies: tan mohair hat, scarf, and mittens. She had to go through every set of drawers and every other possible place to find them.

Without locked doors, people were always coming into Jane's room and taking things or moving them around, especially when she was sleeping. Being in the first room on the right after the central hub, it seemed she had more unwanted visitors than most. This, along with Jane's constant shuffling, meant things never stayed in the same place for any length of time. Relatives were meant to keep the drawers tidy but rarely did, and carers didn't have time, so things tended to end up in a bit of a mess. It always took time to find and sort out any little thing.

Finally, with warm gear in hand, Daisy said, 'OK, Jane, we're all set to go out for the walk. It's a lovely sunny day out there.'

Jane huddled further under the cotton sheets and miserable blanket. Distressed, she said, 'I'm cold.'

Daisy said encouragingly, 'I have all the gear here. You won't be cold outside. You'll be wrapped up warmly.'

Unpersuaded, Jane drew back further into her bed and refused to move.

Used to this routine, Daisy duly sat on the sofa and waited till Jane came around. Morning tea might do it. A nice cuppa, and she was usually ready to go.

Yet it had been uncharacteristically cold this last week. The first week of July, and snow had dumped itself heavily on the Southern Alps, which Daisy could see if she twisted around enough from her seat on the sofa. It was minus three degrees Celsius last night and about the same for the last seven nights.

Daisy was thinking, *Freezing and not heating up much in the day either. We're lucky to get up to ten degrees, and that's only when the sun's out! Twenty degrees is comfort level for humans, probably more for older people. Certainly not that here, much more Arctic.*

Hang on a minute! It's cold in here! I've been here thirty minutes, and I'm still wrapped up in my scarf and padded jacket, and there's Jane still in her thin summer nightie. When she says, 'I'm cold,' she doesn't mean cold outside, which it is, but cold here inside. It's freezing in here!

Seemingly, no one had been getting it. There was no heating in Jane's room – no underfloor heating, no plug for an extra heater in visible sight, certainly no heater anywhere, nothing, no heat-producing anything, nil.

What? Daisy thought. *This is dangerous! Jane's weight is dropping, she has hardly any fat padding as it is with her clothes half falling off her, and here she is in a freezing room!*

Daisy decided to walk around the corridor and check out the other rooms. All the north-facing rooms on Jane's side were cold, except for one where a discerning relative had brought in a good-sized heater and left a big notice near it, saying, 'Turn it on.' Astoundingly, Daisy found that all the south-facing rooms were warm. Underfloor heating, it seemed. *Strange. How can that be? They must know the sun doesn't shine at night.*

And the few miserable rays of north-facing sun that Jane's side got in the day, while welcome, had little flow-on effect to heat the room at night. Concerned, Daisy made enquiries, a number of them. No response.

Finally, she went to the go-to, helpful afternoon nurse who said he would phone up maintenance. Maintenance said, 'We haven't been told to switch on that north-facing side yet.' Unauthorised, the nurse told them to – immediately.

By this time, Jane was frigid. Daisy took her to the near-boiling lounge until she got some colour back in her cheeks. Another cup of tea and a small piece of moist-looking cake, and Jane started to look better already. She would soon have a warm room to go back to, centrally heated with an extra heater as a boost if needed; a daughter had finally bought one in. Perfect. And nice to know her neighbours would be warm now as well.

How long has this deep freeze been going on for? Who knows? No one has been speaking up. Not good. How had no one picked up on this?

Daisy could see the carers were incredibly busy. They hardly had any time for anything as each had nine residents to deal with. They only had time to race in, shower the resident, and then dry and dress them. So they had little time to consider temperature. It was usually hot and steamy from the shower anyway and with all their morning's physical exertion on top of it, with having to lift, hold, and wipe all the way. For them, it was often more like a sauna than the chiller it became later.

Similarly, the cleaning staff were just as busy exerting themselves with heavy vacuum cleaners and other ponderous equipment. They were all warmed up from the effort of having to drag them, so they were not going to notice a bit of chill as anything to worry about.

Laundry staff had just as much on. Briskly bringing in the full set of clothes from yesterday now washed, pressed, and put away neatly (not always) in the residents' drawers and wardrobe, they were there just for a few short moments so wouldn't notice anything like variant temperature levels. Also, the trolley cart those laundry ladies push was massive, a great lump of a thing with thirty lots of residents' laundry teetering on either side. Carting that around would certainly raise temperatures.

So what about the visitors? They must notice. Good question. You would think so except visitors tended to go straight to the main residents' lounge, where it was already warm. So they wouldn't pick up on the room-chiller aspect unless they went to their relative's bedroom to witness it. Most just liked to pop in for a quick visit rather than getting caught up in attending to too much else.

On exiting, they'd quickly drop off the requested shampoo and hair conditioner at the nurses' station rather than walking the extra twenty metres to put it in their mother's bathroom. *Best not to get too involved.* This way, relatives don't get to know anything about the room comfort-wise, view-wise, atmosphere-wise, sun-wise, temperature-wise, facilities-wise, ambience-wise, anything-wise. *Let the nurses look after that. Mum's in good hands. She is well looked after.*

Jane's situation was progressing slowly. Some fronts were better than others. The underfloor heating was on with the extra heater as needed. Good shoes were never purchased, but the velvet slippers sufficed. Medication was stabilised. The chiropodist attended to the bunion, and Jane was now getting a good night's sleep in her own warm room. But Jane was still having problems finding her room, and her walking stride hadn't yet come back.

3

Confidence

'When can I see you?' said the man at the door, courteous enough to at least ask. Others didn't, not getting a very warm reception as a result.

'In a month', said Jane.

Walking back to the sofa, she sat next to Daisy and said, 'I told him in a month, but he won't remember.'

Good negotiation, thought Daisy. Jane was astute, that was for sure. And she had become the most eligible woman in the unit.

Fit at 85, she'd kept her figure from her sporting days. It wasn't long ago that she gave up tennis and golf, and then there were squash and swimming before that and early on skating and gymnastics. Her whole life had been about sport and then, of course, the farm. That was physical, heaving out tussocks and always something to shift or move.

She'd always relied on fitness and strength to compensate for her failings. Being over-medicated had really thrown things out of whack. Again, the endless back and forth with a plethora of similar instructions. 'Stride out so you don't trip. Look for the big red metal roses on the wall, the starting point. Look to the right. Look for the first door on the right, room number 1. Look for your name and room number on the door. Now at your eye level. Jane, room number 1.'

Why was it so difficult to find it? She'd remember for the first few steps, and then she'd forget. Only another twenty steps to go, and she just couldn't get there.

Endless effort. Still, she was used to that from her sporting days. So she didn't mind that side of it. The training was good. It gave her a sense of purpose and achievement, the endless mini-walking track, nurses' station to room and back.

About three times out of nine, she would find the door and enter the room. Three times, she would overshoot and have to be reminded to come back. And in the other three, she would just stand there in the door, saying, 'Am I there yet? Have I made it? Is this it?'

Only once did Daisy hear her say, 'Dear god, I think I've had enough.' Otherwise, never a complaint.

She still had her symptoms to contend with – decreased trunk rotation, slower walking, shorter strides, and ever-shortening steps. Counteracting all these physical limitations would have been overwhelming for most people. But Jane would just say, 'The important thing is achievement. I'm trying to do thoughts to stay on the straight and narrow. It's important not to fritter your life away.'

The other drawback was that, throughout all this, Jane was losing more and more confidence. Considered the most important thing in the training, she'd been proud of her gains. Now she felt she was losing the thread.

When asked if she'd like to go to the lounge, she'd say, 'I'm frightened and not coping. I can't cope being in a group.'

This was in direct contrast to the height of the training back in June when her confidence had peaked, and Daisy asked, 'How confident are you now?'

Jane replied, 'Confident enough.'

'That's about as confident as she gets,' said her daughter, who happened to be standing nearby.

A lot of Jane's confidence at the unit had come from her walking ability. She'd been its fastest and strongest walker by far, always had a spring to her step. Now it was leaden, like the others. Still, ever-conscientious, she kept up the momentum, repeatedly asking, 'What should I be doing next?'

She even said, 'It is fascinating having all these people to work with. I'm feeling a lot better than I was expecting. So many people have gathered around. I have an exciting team.'

Daisy wasn't sure what she meant by this as only the two of them were working with her, so she asked David what he thought. He said, 'She likes to play her part in the team.'

It wasn't always plain sailing. You had to have plenty of patience. Often, 'Got anything interesting?' If not, *I'm going to lie down, but if I don't like what I'm hearing, I'm going to poke my head up.* The lie-downs could often be as much as an hour long, quite a chunk of time, so Daisy would set herself up on the couch and attend to her ever-mounting paperwork. By now, she wasn't just keeping up with and noting Jane's points and progress but she was doing something similar for the thirty other residents as well, albeit a scaled-down version.

Jane took an interest in Daisy's writing and never lost patience with it, which she often did on other things. 'Your work?' she'd say, looking at the notes.

'It's a lot,' said Daisy, at least fifty pages of detailed notes and comments, written in every space. She'd been doing all this for many years now and accrued thousands of pages in the process, keeping up with the residents' comments and expressions so as to notice trends, inconsistencies, threads, interests, capacities, and competencies. It had all to do with their intellectual capacity.

She'd amassed shelves of it, never lost a thing. She prided herself on her filing. Her satchel held a thick stack of papers encased in a clear plastic folder with a good, strong backing board in it and a pen attached. Her favourite set-up, it never left her side.

Nobody ever asked what it was for. All they could see was the writing, writing, writing except Jane's son David. He wanted to know everything. He was incredibly helpful. She could pass stuff by him to have another intellect on board with the work and, importantly, one without dementia. It was critical to get feedback from someone who had an interest and involvement and was keen enough to learn so as to then offer well-informed opinion. Writing was her safe house.

Still thinking about Daisy's writing work, Jane piped up with 'Think of the thrill you are going to get when you get it done.'

Yes, thought Daisy. *A long way to go.*

David was adamant the work had to find a bigger platform. Jane liked to call David on Daisy's cell phone but would often say, 'I won't talk. You say everything.'

When encouraged, it was just, 'How are you, dear?' 'How's the weather?' and 'Has it rained?' Rain was a big factor on the farm.

David, in reply, would say, 'How's the training going, Mum? I hear you're doing well. Keep it up. It's important.'

He was the only one who could de-escalate her mid-tantrum when she'd kicked the table to the other side of the room, with flowers, vase, and food all flying.

Thirty seconds on the phone, and it was, 'All right, I'll try.'

Meanwhile, Daisy kept Jane up to date with what was happening – the doctor's visits, changes in medication, family meetings. To it all, she'd say, 'I'm interested, and I want to understand.'

She wasn't, though, invited to the family meeting with the doctor, them all discussing her health, which Daisy didn't agree with, but it was how the other three siblings wanted it. Jane was left in her room, saying, 'I hope they're going to include me in on anything that happens to me.'

It didn't look promising. David had asked Daisy to keep Jane company while they were in the meeting so she didn't feel left out. Of course, she would have felt a lot less left out if she was actually in the meeting rather than outside it, but David wasn't the POA (his sister was) so didn't have full power to negotiate. He'd already pushed for the notes. That was mission enough.

Jane's room orientation was getting better, and she could find her room at least half the time now. Still, the mind-training work was episodic. Often, she'd say, 'I don't want to do anything. It's a pull because I have to concentrate.' It was only after a lie-down on the bed that she seemed to be able to recalibrate enough to then continue.

Then once up, it was, 'What's next?' And she was into it again.

Aiming to get her better socialised with the residents in the lounge, Daisy would take her there for walks, Jane now agreeing to go there. Sometimes they would sit with one or two other residents to ease her into low-key socialisation.

On one such occasion, they sat next to Janet and Warren, both regulars at the workshops. Warren had a warm and engaging personality; Janet was more severe, but you could see Jane liked her clipped approach, not unlike her own. Warren said, 'You feel better being a part of it.'

Hearing that Jane had sore knees, he said, 'You have to be well to take the benefit, or the pain keeps coming to the fore.'

Daisy was spending extra voluntary time with Jane to accommodate her sleeps and low moods. This way, they could at least get something constructive from each session. Jane said, 'I haven't had much support.'

'It must be great feeling the support now,' said Daisy.

'Yes, psychologically', she said. 'I hope you and David can feel my appreciation.' Jane seemed to recalibrate herself with the bed relaxation. She always got up more invigorated and settled.

The discussions they had were often philosophical in nature, Daisy still having to be careful not to overload Jane with questions. But on one especially good day, she asked, 'What can you see through the eyes?'

'Love', said Jane.

'And what does a depressed person need?'

'Peace.'

'Do you know what I think?'

'I hate to think.'

'You have a good intellect, Jane. That was a bright answer.'

'I hope so.'

'It's good to accept a compliment.'

When being taken to lunch, Jane would often say, 'I don't want to go. I have my friend here. Put it in my room or heat it up later.'

Staff felt they'd accommodated enough of Daisy's extended escapades and started pulling the plug. They told Daisy to cut her voluntary time, saying it was 'too much' for Jane. Quickly seeing the danger zone ahead with reduced availability, Daisy had to up the ante with Jane. So she said, 'It's time now that you have to come to the workshops.' David supported her.

The timing worked well. Jane came, and as long as the topics were to her interest, most of the time, she'd attend. Fortunately, her interests were in tune with the other residents'. Most of them were on a similar par, though Jane was now one step ahead from all her private sessions with Daisy. Confidence continued to be their favourite theme, that and how to settle the fuzzy, racing mind.

Jane excelled. She gave well-framed answers and often led the discussion. This was a big step up from the perfunctory 'good morning' and 'good evening' to the residents set at her dining table. 'I feel I'm getting a more conscious mind, and you don't growl at me, which is a plus,' she said. Her confidence was growing.

Now that her private lessons were much reduced, she would have to find her way in the crowd to make things work for her. She'd started talking to staff, so that was a step forward. One afternoon a tall Indian carer from Bangalore was taking her to dinner. As they passed the nurses' station, Daisy overheard Jane saying, 'Am I having my training?'

Daisy updated the carer, to which Jane said, 'So there's hope.'

Later, Jane told Daisy, 'We didn't really realise what we had got ourselves in for. Or I didn't. When you look back on all the things we have done, we've have done well. It's a big ask for anybody.'

4

Keep Calm

Daisy enjoyed working with the residents. That was the easy part. The Filipino carers were a delight as well. With some, that was where it often stopped.

Once such carers got their New Zealand nursing registration, everything changed. Now promoted as the new elite, they amply applied it full force. 'You are not a physiotherapist here!'

'Don't even think about it.'

'Don't take her down the stairs. We'll lose our nursing licence.'

'Keep her on the walker.'

'It doesn't matter what you think. That's not important.'

Daisy knew full well the resident could walk ably on her own. She had good stability and balance. She was walking fine. In fact, the walker was more of a hazard than anything. It was a nightmare.

It seemed the only ones she could have a laugh with were the residents.

Bullying was rife and often directed towards her. Being tall and white, she hardly blended into the scenery. It had always worked in her favour up to this point but now seemingly not. She'd always had positive feedback for her work, getting good results on most occasions, but here, it wasn't the work but toeing the line that was important. Quick march!

Hauled into the office by the unit manager, Daisy was under review. 'I have had a complaint from one of the relative talking about confidence,' she said.

'Confidence is for children when their brains are still growing, not adults. You are not to talk to the residents about confidence. And don't talk to them about memory. They have none, and it will never come back!'

After this vociferous download, Daisy said, 'How about some commendations? All you ever do is criticise.'

'You try commendations in a country with a hundred million people and see how that works,' she said stiffly. Daisy was too big for her boots. She needed to be pulled down a peg or two.

It was not like this with the residents. They liked Daisy and told her so. She, in turn, felt the same.

Workshops benefited both parties. Quickly, a mutual admiration society developed. The residents were brilliant as far as Daisy was concerned. Of course, they were rock bottom on confidence, heads down most of the time, hardly saying a thing. She'd be heading that way too if she succumbed to the barrage she was getting. But when they did speak, it had such depth and insight. Well worth the wait.

With all the workshops, she'd give them a range of topics to choose from, anything from reducing stress, being positive, or how to improve one's thinking capacity. They loved the lot, confidence themes being the favourite. She'd been reading up on positive psychology, lots of depth and detail. That made the topics easy to speak to.

What to do if being criticised was the first workshop. *Apt*, thought Daisy, *well experienced at this point*.

'Talk it through,' said Gwen.

Difficult, thought Daisy.

'Retreat', said Trisha. Certainly what Daisy felt like doing.

'A rough response is not the answer,' replied Warren.

'You have to stop and think about what you are saying. Otherwise, it won't be what you really want to say. Sum it up before saying anything, very important. We are saying and doing wrong all the time,' said Jane.

Wise words, thought Daisy. *Think before you speak*. She'd try harder.

There was stress in the unit. You could cut the air with a knife. Workshops were going against the status quo, ruffling feathers big time. 'Daisy, are you following the monthly calendar? Three o'clock, time for games.'

Games, thought Daisy. *Here, this woman has hardly uttered a word. She has just found confidence to say something, and you want me to throw her a tennis ball in the midst of it. How to throw cold water on progress, that is what these games should be called.*

Still, Daisy wasn't going to give up, not now. Too much water had passed under the bridge. She kept stretching time frames, saying, 'Yes, yes, I will.' She still managed to get the residents' comments noted down.

Counteracting stress was the next topic. Again, apt. Jane was leading the way with 'You have to consider everything. Be positive. Think of what the opposition are thinking.'

Janet said, 'Sort it out. Be calm. Think differently.'

And Warren stated, 'You need to sort it out.'

Exactly, thought Daisy. *No need to fork out thousands on New Age remedies when you can get the wisdom pearls right here.*

The residents had an incredible range of life experience, all through the war and depression. They'd learnt the hard way. People should be queuing up to hear them.

Looking to the right, Daisy could see the nurse poking her head imperiously over the computer. *Will they never give up? Where did they get that army discipline?*

No doubt, management higher-up were bearing down on them, asking for reports on the recalcitrant Daisy; one nurse said, 'We have been asked to look over you.' Ratcheting up. Heavens above!

It was serious stuff, ridiculous if it wasn't for the fact that her job was under threat because of it and, with that, all the work they were doing. She wasn't going to leave the residents high and dry, and she didn't want to leave their thinking work half-formed either. She knew this group had the most to offer. If she lost ground at this point, she'd never get it back, too difficult.

The stress of announced surveillance was getting a bit beyond the pale. She was almost at the point of getting in her lawyer friends. Discussing it with them, one said, 'That's ridiculous. Don't they realise confidence is what it is all about?'

'That's a good way to dampen enthusiasm, isn't it? What qualification does the unit manager have to speak about confidence? She is too opinionated. Is she a psychologist? You are a professional.'

'It's not in your contract what you should speak about.'

'She should have said, "Look, that relative is stressed. Steer clear of her when she is around."'

The other lawyer said, 'Can they do this?'

'Yes, if a complaint is made', came the reply.

'Say you'll take your lawyer to the next meeting.'

Residents weren't aware of all these goings-on, not early on anyway. They had little capacity for it. They'd only just started to think about things themselves.

One thing that did click with them, though, was Daisy's humour. She'd morphed it a bit by listening to old footage of Aunt Daisy's 1950s radio show, of which they were all firm adherents, their national icon. Start the day off with singing 'Daisy Daisy' and away they'd go.

'We oldies always like to have fun,' said Gabrielle. Allegiance right there. Fun they were having, Daisy included. She could feel herself loosening up. It was doing her good.

Having always been good at telling a joke and stories along with it, she'd found the Aunt Daisy persona pretty easy to emulate. Starting off with 'Good morning. Good morning, everybody.' Then it was news of the week, news of the world, history of the world. That pretty much summed it up. All was good as long as told with currency, enthusiasm, and humour.

Residents were still not saying much, but they were certainly becoming good at listening and laughing – halfway there, totally out of their depth. The staff had no idea what was going on. They didn't get the humour and couldn't see why anyone would laugh at it.

Daisy had unwittingly found the holy grail. Under Aunt Daisy, she could get away with practically anything. No staff would report back to management when they didn't know the context. She was starting to enjoy it, that being the whole point of it.

From there on in, things kept moving forward. Drawing on the Kiwi culture was having the fortuitous effect of revitalising reality for the residents, building it back brick by brick. Residents were now concentrating and contributing, definitely thinking. Daisy could see the computation.

'You come away thinking differently to varying degrees each time. Rather than letting things slip, you start thinking so you can reassess everything,' said Jane.

And Helena said, 'There were always several things to think about after the workshops.'

Then it was courage and confidence. 'Keep going. Keep quiet. Keep your distance,' said Deidre, a solo mother and former nurse.

Exactly, thought Daisy. *What I'll have to learn if ever I get to tell this tale.*

It was difficult having been an extrovert all her life. The staff here were perfect at it, quiet as mice. You'd have five in the room, working like mad. And you'd hardly know they were there.

Staff management was still very much centred on a command-and-control culture. Daisy found it oppressive. The other tasks she was being asked to do she was hopeless at. Serving lunch for thirty? She'd never been a waitress. Serving drinks at happy hour? She didn't even drink. How was she to know what went with what? Anyway, she had no interest in it, and she couldn't see the point. How was it relevant for residents? Ridiculous in her view. They'd all had to give up everything on entering, drinking and smoking included. So why tantalise with one miserable drink on a Saturday afternoon pitched as the latest cordon bleu creation? She couldn't do it. Unless harassed, she would wait until the next round. The residents didn't want alcohol anyway. She'd already asked them. That was the last thing on their minds.

Deidre's advice to 'keep going, keep quiet, and keep your distance', Daisy was implementing poorly. Rattled by ever-present surveillance (didn't they realise this was not the way to do things to get the best from their staff?), the trolley of drinks somehow found its way flying through the stratosphere and crashing head first onto the floor. No idea how that happened, an equation of physics in there somewhere. She was now damaging property into the bargain. If she came out of this unharmed, it was going to take some doing.

The one and only thing that was working well at this point was the workshops. Residents came to them all, committed, full effort. They were admirable.

'We need a confident presenter,' said Jane. The group assented, nodding, saying they considered Daisy such. So buoyed by that new-found appreciation, she once again found herself acknowledging its power.

Daisy could see the residents' thinking capacity growing. Depth and detail was sharpening, and the comments they were contributing were analytical and well thought out. Still, though, they weren't communicating with one another freely. No one was taking the initiative. Except for the odd one-liners at the dinner table, it was really just perfunctory communication, no self-starter conversations yet.

Daisy was beginning to wonder if it would ever happen. She knew they had the intelligence for it. That was obvious. But it must have been the confidence they were missing and having no role model amidst them doing the same. They conversed well in the workshops, but it was mainly with Daisy and the whiteboard, not with one another. And staff weren't encouraging it. They didn't even think they could think, let alone read or converse, though that changed later down the track. It had to happen naturally somehow. Daisy just hoped she'd be there to witness it.

The day arrived, 10 August 2018. She came through the door, and there they were, the three of them. They'd pulled up the chairs to the bay windows and were having a good old chat after breakfast. It had happened – of their own volition entirely. Warren was the one to have pulled over the chairs, being the strongest amongst the three. But they were talking, all right. Daisy could not just see them but also hear them from the nurses' station. She knew this was going to be the starting point of something much greater.

It didn't take long, and the whole place was humming. It was that first role model, amidst themselves, that they needed. In the next few months, the window bays were packed. Everyone was keen to have a chat in the sun, with one another. Good company, background music, cup of tea – what could be nicer? One of their greatest joys in life had returned.

From then on, progress escalated. Their communing improved confidence, vocabulary, word usage, and articulation. They were all learning big time. Into the light, making friends, giving their opinions, testing the waters – community had started. The second group of residents who came into the unit were to be far more assertive and articulate than this first group, having the advantage of a developing community to step right into.

5

Using Their Intellect

Theodora arrived at the unit. She was a real force, a quantum leap in articulation. The other ladies had only just started to converse, and here she was, having intelligible conversations, refusing to accept anything wrong with her. 'What dementia? Well, I don't have it!'

She went about getting her room sorted, bossing everyone around. Arranging the magazines and books she'd bought in, she made sure her handy sidekick walker was within peripheral view. If taken, she'd swiftly wrap the thief over both knuckles in quick succession, curbing a second try.

She disassociated herself from the less able and would only communicate with you if you looked well off or well schooled as she'd been. Acerbic and quick with a sarcastic wit, you'd have to wonder why she was there.

Direction orientation – she could go to her room a hundred times, and she still wouldn't remember it. She never complained; she hardly got out. Her family had visited little. Constricted and confined, she just said, 'Have to make the best of a bad situation.'

She was always busy reading and got perturbed when she saw others dozing off. 'Some people here sleep a lot,' she said in an accusatory tone.

'It's often because they're sick or medicated,' said Daisy, hoping to arouse some sympathy.

'Well, you'd think they could become interested in something,' she'd say while flicking through the latest *Vogue*.

The half-sleeping ladies now woke up groggily with painful cricks in the neck, no complaints. Neck pain was way down the list of their unwanted problems, certainly compared with physio waiting rooms where Daisy had worked. There, it was rated top priority.

With the newspaper reading about to start, Theodora said imperiously, 'But I can read the paper myself. I don't need the paper read to me.'

'Yes, but not everyone here is able,' Daisy would reply for the umpteenth time.

It was the same every morning. She never let up, no mercy for the fact that others had less ability than her. She liked the already intelligent. 'I want a man,' she'd say, 'intelligent and not ugly.' One way or another, in her eyes, she was going to get it.

Exasperating in the extreme, she was nevertheless important to the group. She raised the bar of what was possible. One bridge-building gesture she achieved, heroic in the light of present memory loss, was getting to know everyone's names. This was after a lot of questioning and considerable personal effort. Daisy wasn't sure if this was for the advancement of ego or social relations, but either way, it was proving a point. It was possible.

Residents were aghast. It could have gone either way. Shut down and shut off or rise to the challenge? Fortunately, a few decided to up the ante, a brave move as their vocabulary was only a fraction of hers. But with Daisy being the backup dictionary, the train was on its way.

She was still battling away with her trusty whiteboard, no advanced technology yet. It was a momentous task getting a range of topics as enticing as when Hamlet burst onto the scene. It took a week's research to get the depth and detail they liked, all put into a show-like format for best entertainment value.

The discerning audience, though limited in memory, certainly had their opinions. As Janice, a former university lecturer in accountancy, said, 'It must have something in it.'

Daisy became the sole producer of these hefty monologues – researcher, producer, narrator, and actor all in one. This way, they could interrupt, ask questions, get more detail, keep up with the plot, slow it down, stop it, restart it, all in tune with their learning ability and the numerous goings-on at the unit.

After a week of intense preparation and the subject sorted, Theodora would quiz, 'Well, what is it? Tell me.'

If the topic didn't appeal, she'd quickly reject with a dismissive wave. 'Don't like that.'

Daisy had to backpedal fast to get support from everyone. Without it, things went flat, and there was no uptake. It was all about psyche and preparation, but once the right topic and approach was struck, the watershed was worth it.

Daisy's biggest inspiration came from the residents themselves saying they liked it. 'We like to think.'

'We like to learn.'

'We're doing our best.'

'We're trying hard.' They definitely were. Daisy could see it.

In this pioneering time, Marjorie arrived at the unit. A wealthy spinster from an aristocratic family, she had been brought up in one of William and Dorothy Wordsworth's houses in the Lake District. A host of golden daffodils, and yes, she could recite it.

As hawk-eyed as ever and never missing a beat, Marjorie wouldn't deign to sit in the group but would listen inquisitively from afar. After some months of such inquisition, she pulled Daisy aside and said in her upper-class English accent, 'Good work, good education. It is good to learn something.'

Well, that has to be the best endorsement to date, thought Daisy, as she was an astute national physiotherapy examiner from her physio days.

Maintaining the interest of the residents was the hardest part. They fortunately, by now, were coming up with ever-more-insightful ways to hold on to their mercurial concentration. 'Follow your line of thought through,' said Helena.

'Make up your own mind,' said Jane.

'You can be disciplined when you come to a conclusion in your own mind as you have more conviction. You need to be convinced,' Janet said astutely in her clipped, manicured voice.

Though it was slow and would take weeks of workshops to get these bejewelled one-liners out, Daisy could see the overall thinking capacity and confidence growing. Some days were better than others.

Over time, Daisy was able to read their state of mind just by noting their expressions. When the racing dementia mind kicked in, the character quickly changed – smile gone, warmth evaporated and a much more serious expression, fight-and-flight mode personified, often rapidly spiralling into reactive ranting and raving as supposed sundowner hits. Otherwise, when thinking through their intellect and using their intelligence actively, they were relaxed and at ease, readily smiling with expressive faces, bright eyed with warm, engaging expressions. If Daisy could catch them in the early triggering, spiralling stages, she could sometimes help in turning them round, if she could maintain the resident's trust and interest enough to make the effort to do so.

Daphne, a former nurse with glorious blue eyes, had two daughters who rarely visited; and when they did, she had a hard job recognising them. Still, she had a remarkable ability to keep upbeat. Never depressed, she was always alert and bright eyed, taking everything in, full surveillance, 360 degrees. Noticing her keen observation skills, Daisy approached her and asked what it was she was viewing.

'It looks to me as if they are thinking,' Daphne said.

'Oh, excellent.' So this was her new interest, looking to see if others were thinking. Now that was something!

She also had another skill as subtle as the first, working away with her eyes, which were like those of the actress Amy Adams. Something seemed to be going on in there. Ever forward, Daisy asked again what she was doing, and Daphne said with her dry Irish humour, 'I'm taking your power.' No joke. You could see and feel her doing just that, not in a vampirish sort of way but in a 'well, I need it, and you have it, so it's OK then' sort. She'd draw Daisy over and say she wanted to look at her. Then she'd bring her head down to her eye level and clamp on, energy drawing. It was a fascinating exercise, one she'd devised herself. Irish eyes were smiling literally.

When Daisy went to see Daphne at the hospital after she had a fall in her room and fractured her hip, her enquiring eyes were just the same, radiating iridescent ocean blue. Daisy admired her developing her own self-empowering methods, effectively rising above her severe immobility issues and family disinterest. She'd been a joy to many, and you'd always remember their contribution.

The residents were working hard, and the more they worked, the more the lounge took on a level-headed, literati calm, intelligence at work. Their interest developed their concentration. The concentration developed their focus. And the focus built their confidence.

Still, though, for some, the effort of the concentration required was extremely difficult. Some were saying, 'I don't want to do anything as it's too hard to concentrate.'

There were other challenges as well. The background din was ever present – clattering in the kitchen, chattering at the nurses' station, the ever-present medication trolley doing its three-times-a-day rounds. *How do these residents here cope?* Daisy thought. After eight hours, her ears were ringing. Goodness only knows what it was like to be here 24/7.

'Can you keep the noise down?' Theodora would shout out. But staff were time compressed, and throwing the dishes wholesale into the dishwasher was far faster than silently putting them away one by one.

*   *   *

Theodora was the first to make it known she could partake ably in crosswords. The first three she answered that Daisy witnessed were from a giant women's weekly quiz:

A wreath of flowers and leaves (7) (a garland)

Building with a circular interior and plan, especially with a dome (7) (a rotunda)

Celtic tribe of which Boudicca was queen (5) (Iceni)

Jack, a new arrival, got:

Animals which were part of Carthage's army in battles against Rome (9) (elephants)

The claw of a bird of prey (5) (talon)

Tapering four-sided stone pillar set up as a monument or landmark (7) (obelisk)

So neck and neck, they had each answered three. You could see Theodora's ears pricking up. A challenge had arrived. They'd hardly met, and she was already saying publicly she enjoyed Jack's intellectual stimulation. He probably did hers as well, though he was much more contained with his utterances.

'Learning is communication, which is education. You can absorb knowledge from another person. A lot of people can lose their power of thinking,' says Jack.

'You have to get people thinking. That's what we are short of here, information. It's a big thing to impart news and knowledge to other people and have the vocabulary to do it.'

Theodora was eyeing him up. He had, after all, nearly beaten her in the crossword. She was now saying of Jack, 'He accepts it.'

'What?' said Daisy.

'His smartness. He thinks he's pretty smart. He's good at expressing himself, and he uses his intelligence to his best advantage.'

'It's the way you use your smartness. Keeping your train of thought is a big thing. You have to keep going,' Jack responded.

Jack didn't spend much time in the lounge, so Theodora didn't get to talk to him as much as she would like. Even when he did come in, he sat way back in the dining room, which was just about as bad as not being there at all. Still, she'd find a way around it somehow.

Meanwhile, she was making a friend of Delilah, another schoolteacher with a similar background. Well spoken and quiet with a panache for good manners, she suited Theodora down to the ground. A card arrived for Delilah in elegant handwriting, which she had difficulty reading. She duly handed it to Theodora. It was from a good friend sending condolences for the death of Delilah's husband. Staff didn't realise it had got through the system. Reference to people dying was generally kept hush-hush.

Theodora read and reread the card to Delilah in a sympathetic manner, consoling her more than any staffer would have likely done had they read it. This was the first initiative of any conciliatory individual interaction of note Daisy had seen. It was a positive sign.

She was aware the residents needed breathing space and reflection time, to digest such news and to be able to think things through quietly by themselves. After dinner, and the news was the ideal time. It was decided a night programme would be set up.

Bach and Beethoven were put on at seven, and the residents could just sit back and relax, transported to their favourite place. Amidst this serenading, a selection of magazines was also offered, like air hostesses of old, so they'd have something to flick through. One generous and understanding relative, whose mother had now gone to the hospital, came in and gave Daisy not only her own stack of women's weekly magazines but her friends' recent piles as well. It was an armload. They were good quality, near brand new, latest gossip, scrumptious. These generous gestures from relatives made all the difference as there was very little reading at the unit (usually just the favourite books of the deceased) and certainly no new stuff coming in except for the one and only daily newspaper.

After one such delivery and armed with Meghan and Harry's latest escapades, Daisy decided to give them to Theodora to be the librarian. She asked if she could share them with the other ladies. 'Oh yes, of course.' She'd be delighted.

'Would Beverly [Jack's wife] like a magazine?' Theodora called out.

'No, she doesn't read,' Jack replied. He hadn't even considered the possibility.

'Would you like a magazine?' Theodora called again, this time addressing Beverly.

'Yes', came the reply. Yes, she would like it. And yes, she would read it.

'Oh yes, she can flick the pages over,' said Jack.

If not for Theodora's quick thinking, Beverly could have easily missed out.

This new nightly routine was suiting Theodora perfectly, better than rugby blaring away. As she had been saying for ages, 'We shouldn't be so regimented. We need some free time for reading.'

After her first evening conversation with Jack, she was saying with full entitlement, 'It's nice to sit next to a man and have an intelligent conversation.'

'Anyway, it's all going quite well, isn't it?'

6

Thwarted

Jack arrived at the unit, looking immaculate, well shaven, smartly dressed, and definitely dapper. 'All the training, thirty years in the army.' Most stayed for seven.

Jack demanded little of his environment not because of a lack of resources but because he liked it that way, spartan, just like the barracks. 'Makes you think better.' He lived and breathed it. The military had taught him most of what he knew, and he thrived on it.

Barracks were great. Food was fine, uniforms smart. There was nothing about it that he complained about. That way, you kept upbeat. No complaints.

He kept his thinking good. He thought a lot. And he had quite a range. He gave credit to his intellectual prowess to the army. 'I had to use my brain and memory all through my military life. I was being educated all through that time – promotion examinations, trade examinations, gunnery, radio, armoured vehicle driving and maintenance, then having to instruct others. Keeps your mind active, having to impart knowledge to others in the unit. You are virtually a teacher of military affairs. Your mind is always being used. Your powers of thinking in the military really increase as there is so much to learn and do. You don't vegetate.' Thinking, he could take you right back to Mesopotamia, the Tigris and Euphrates, all the military history, and forwards right through to rockets and global warming. He was sharp, and he liked to keep it that way.

Jack's a great advocate of the elderly and their problems. He can reiterate lengthy transcripts from just a few questions, a neat compilation of insights and hard-earned observations.

Jack did, though, have memory problems, present-day ones. Every morning Jack would come up to the nurses' desk distressed. 'Where's my razor? Have you seen it? My razor?'

On occasions, staff lost patience. How many times did they have to explain? 'Yes, the razor was safe, above the sink beside the toothbrush, where it had always been.'

Witnessing this tirade, Daisy called Jack over. 'Jack, you're an intelligent man. But your present memory is not good. You have to find a way to work around this. Not being able to find your razor is because of your faded memory. Find a way, and you'll reduce your stress.'

'OK', Jack said. 'I'll forget about it. Doesn't matter. I'll grow a beard if I have to.' He never mentioned it again.

Now he was not immaculately shaved, certainly not like the army. But he was bright as a button on all other accounts, having carved out quite a role for himself at the unit.

Jack was the only man there with his wife. Beverly was a professional tennis coach. She wore stretchy black and white checked pants and cheerful orange jackets. Few women could get away with it. But they suited her. A self-contained person with a wry sense of humour, she didn't mind Jack's avid socialising. 'I don't mind,' she said dourly. 'He's always been like that.'

It took Jack a good half an hour to go the full thirty metres from his bedroom to the lounge. Meeting and greeting was important business. Mrs Choo was the first to put her hands out, chattering away in some Chinese dialect; he can't understand a thing. He gave lots of handshakes, nods, and little pats on the back of the hand with made-up Chinese if he had to.

The women in the unit crave men's company. Most of their husbands had died, so Jack's attention was always well received. The nurses' station was where the escalated women gathered with their perpetual 'When can I get out?' and 'Why can't I get home?' laments. A gentle pat on the shoulder from the 'conveniently passing' Jack and a 'This is your home, dear. This is where we all live now' generally quelled the cries faster than any staffer can manage. And it was genuine. Jack understood their plight. He was right in there with them after all. But he was well reconciled to the fact that this was his 'last posting'.

When the men wailed, 'I don't want to die,' he simply said, 'We have to die sometime, mate. And none of us are going to get out of here alive. So you better accept it.' And they did. His pragmatic 'sergeant major' approach to the men and 'supportive mentor' to the women worked wonders. All good so far.

So entered Marina, a real minx. Feline in looks with all the acquired attributes, she used them to the max. Long slim legs that reached to her waist and a face that elongated to the chin, she was certainly vampish; you'd have to give her that.

Hardly able to string two words together, she was only articulate when cursing, generally to women who got in her way. Not one to use her intellect and having no intention of doing so, she nevertheless preferred intelligent men. That meant Jack and David would be the unwitting targets. Let's see who had the strength to resist her.

First, David. She was snaking around him, full-body lean and unabashedly sliding her arm into his, hands intertwined, head leaning softly into his shoulder. David was incensed. 'My Suzy !' he cried. 'I love Suzy .'

David was a good-looking tall former detective. Suzy, his wife, had always been a supportive partner. Marina, knowing David was married, still stalked, unabashed. David, often beside himself with not knowing how to get rid of her, was frequently rescued by staff and taken to the safety of the locked nurses' station. Doing jigsaw puzzles to get his mind off things, he actually enjoyed his new-found domain.

Well, she can't climb over the nurses' station (probably could, leggy enough). Let's go for Jack.

In full view of Beverly, she slunk right in. Jack was sitting straight as a statue, immobile, purring, mesmerised.

Daisy was appalled. This woman had something. What was it? She didn't want to look too hard unless she came under her corrupt spell as well. Had she mastered hypnosis?

They tried to get her to move from Jack; it was a resounding 'no!' After being explained that Jack was married, she said, 'Doesn't matter.' After they tried to tease them apart, she just went for a full-on cat cling. Daisy was clearly exasperated.

'Getting frustrated, are we?' said an amused David, pleased he was out of the fray but couldn't resist the dig.

Something had to be done. This woman was something else. And she was cruel. Daisy had witnessed it. She'd put out an unflinching foot, tripping up the less able residents. Then if questioned, he would say, 'They deserve it.'

Concerned relatives, seeing partners go down, were just given convenient platitudes of 'It's the dementia.' Daisy didn't think so. She was a mean minx. She knew exactly what she was doing. You don't learn these skills from dementia, no way.

Still thinking on how to approach it all, Daisy had to take the exercise class. Everyone was there, full force. Marina, mincing away and darting eyes all around, was ready for the next pounce. No conscience, she locked on with formidable sensualist stares. *That woman really knows how to use her eyes*, thought Daisy, *and in all the wrong ways*. Vaudevillian on the one hand, disarming and charming on the other.

She looked at Jack, now the latest statuary. Aiming to get her off balance, Daisy had to give her something. So she let her come to the front, performing being Marina's favoured ritual, which of course she did ably, hip rolling and conniving, outflanking Daisy as the exercise trainer in an instant.

Then something totally unexpected happened. Daisy unwittingly turned into a full-on sergeant major. 'All right, sit down, Marina!' she barked. 'Now! And you, Jack, sit by your wife. And, David, stay there and don't move. And, Marina, you stay there and definitely don't move. And I mean ever! Stay where you are, all of you!'

Shock. Silence. Pause.

'He's got his hand on hers. I'm going to change that,' machinated Marina under her sultry breath, referring to Jack and Beverly.

'You will not be doing anything of the sort, Marina. And I mean anything! You are going to leave these men alone and give them some privacy!'

Struck at her own performance and the assembled forces' compliance, Daisy could feel the endorphins rise. She could see the gobsmacked charge staff in her peripheral vision. Jack was also smiling. 'Just like in the army.'

Amassing all her control, Daisy de-escalated somewhat by saying, 'Now stay this way, and I'll see you all at nine o'clock tomorrow morning!'

She thought later that a good ending would have been, 'You are dismissed', but thought better of it.

Daisy could see the charge nurse smiling. Medication rounds didn't generally provide this sort of entertainment.

Doing her notes at the front desk, Daisy considered Jack had got the message, not so Marina. She walked past, muttering just loud enough to be heard, 'I still look younger than all those other women.' She believed she was a cut above. She'd rival Joan Collins if she had a chance. Mid-eighties meant nothing. Conniving, she was as clear as a bell. Otherwise, hardly a word she said made sense.

Daisy didn't want to think about it too much, but was it something to do with criminal intelligence? Maybe Marina being challenged was making her think. She was certainly speaking more clearly. Whatever, Daisy didn't want her corrupting attitude disrupting the residents' lives and disrupting her work. She was a real handful.

The others were fine. Jack was sorted, Beverly reassured, and David at ease. It was then dinner, the news, supper, and lights out.

Day to day, Beverly continued to be stoic and dour. She had a dry sense of humour, but it took a certain something to get it going. Having been brought up on a large sheep farm with three brothers and no sisters, she preferred and felt more comfortable in male company.

Beverly and Jack had led independent lives, he in the army, she as a coach. Now they were together 24/7. You could see Jack was getting frustrated. He knew Beverly was deteriorating, but why did she have to open and close that top button on her shirt all the time? 'Bev, stop that,' he'd say loudly. Of course, they were not in the privacy of their own home now, were they. Thirty sets of straining ears hardly made it that. Giving him no response, a common practice on her part, she carried on doing exactly what she was doing. Jack, frustrated, went to his room.

He continued the 'Morning, Bev,' at the start of each day and greeted her at every meal. He still referred to her as his wife and always looked out for her if anyone started to abuse her. It was difficult, though, when there was no conversation and so little response to anything he said. And these minxes prowling around him weren't making it any easier.

There had been some impact after Daisy's tirade. Marina slunk around with her tail between her legs, and the men had a well-earned break from her advances. Everyone could take a breather for a couple of days.

The next week, though, Marina was at it again. Daisy tried moving her. No such luck. She clung onto Jack like a shipwreck victim, too dramatic for words. And David was chiming to Daisy, 'You're intimated!' Again, unhelpful.

In the end, Daisy went to Beverly and asked if she wanted to see Jack. 'Yes', she said. Good. Back to Jack, Daisy delivered the verdict. Conscience kicking in, 'I better go back,' he said.

Marina was outwitted. 'Oh, no', she said, launching into profanities.

*   *   *

Daisy came to work after her break. Staff said Jack wasn't getting out of bed. He'd just lie there all day, hardly getting up for meals. *What? What's happening?* Daisy thought. She promptly went to his room.

Seeing him lying prostrate on the bed, she retorted, 'What's happening?'

'I'm tired,' he said, 'getting old.'

'I'm sorry, Jack, but you can't be getting tired and old, lying down here on your bed all day, not now, not ever. What are all the people here going to do? You are needed out there.

It's important. You can't just lie down here and do nothing. It's no good for you or anyone else. You have to get up and support yourself!'

'All right', he said and, without much further ado, got up charged, potent, and adrenalised. Quick smart, that was the end of that! Henceforth, he theorised, hypothesised, and intellectualised, often sharing his thoughts with Daisy at the end of her workday.

Jack's son came to visit, not a common occurrence as he lived in Australia. He took Jack and Beverly out, and they had a lovely day. 'Jack's always been super-intelligent. He has a different disease to Beverly. She has Alzheimer's, brain rot. I wish I had a tablet of what he's on,' he said.

Jack was now up and about. Joining in more activities now, he was sorely realising he too could slide, just like the best of them. He was not as invincible as he thought.

The Crown was now on, the residents' favourite. Netflix was never more appreciated. 'Ooh, I love it. The actors are so good. How they play their parts,' cooed Theodora.

'Insight into royal living', quipped Jack. 'The Queen is just a human being, just more privileged. I've met her, held her commission in the army.'

'What?' the group said in obvious awe. 'You've met the Queen!'

'Shaken her hand.'

'You'll never want to wash your hand again!' they chorused in timely admiration.

'I can imagine you, Jack, in all that regalia,' crooned Theodora, now making no bones of the fact that, while looking for a man, she considered Jack the most eligible.

It was awkward for him, being married to Beverly. And of course, he had just got over his recent Marina sink. Can't afford to go through that again.

'You must be pretty important,' Theodora said, taking her chance.

'That's right,' said Jack. 'I'm not a cabbage!'

'Should we call you sir and bow?'

Unperturbed, he explained, 'It's a powerful gesture. Bowing and saluting are a formal gesture of respect and courtesy.'

'Can you do one for us?'

Jack stood and gave a full military salute, military and naval. 'Naval salute has the back of the hand facing forward rather than the palm as it often has tar on it from waterproofing the boats.'

Then it was deft demonstrations of drawing a weapon. Still slim and statuesque in the women's eyes, these swift manoeuvres, all for their benefit, were clearly heroic. 'If you are right-handed, you have your sword or pistol on the left so you can draw it across your body, like this!' Jack snappily demonstrated.

'Yes, we are learning so much, aren't we?' said Theodora.

'Yes, we love to learn,' the group chorused.

Soon after the salute and sword demonstration, Daisy noticed Jack was sitting excessively straight in the central back row. *Like Tutankhamen*, she thought, *self-consciously so. What was up this time?*

Beverly was sitting to Jack's left, but there, too, was the subtly scheming Theodora. She had worked her way surreptitiously onto his right. 'Will you hold my hand?' she'd said beseechingly.

Jack was stuck between a rock and a hard place. Not wanting to offend and not wanting to burn any bridges either (they may be needed to scuttle across later), he had tentatively placed his hands birdlike on both sets. Daisy looked around. She seemed to be the only one to have noticed.

7

Daisy Interviews Jack

Daisy believes that if she was able to interview Jack the conversation may well have gone as follows...

Given that so many insights which only those with dementia, who also have a high level of thinking, possess.

Daisy: How do you keep so sharp?

Jack: Life becomes very iffy when you get older. Men retire at 65 and then just become cabbages. The mind goes into retirement as well. It's difficult to make relationships as you don't know how long they are going to last. You can't make plans as you don't know if you will see them come to fruition. So you can only plan from day to day.

You have to be a lot sharper and listen to what others say to get an outside view of what's going on. You have to have a brighter mind to manage your own life. If you lose it, you can't manage.

You have to be interesting. You have to keep up with political affairs and current affairs to make yourself interesting and keep your mind alive. Anything interesting in the newspaper, you can bring up. Anything in your past life, that's relevant. Automatically then, there will be integration with everyone. If not, you won't be interesting to talk to, and no one will want to talk to you.

You have to have a good knowledge of what's going on around you. If you have nothing to talk about, you can't communicate. Magazines, TV, glitzy stuff can take over. You have to be careful not to fill up on cabbage information. That's just filling up with nothing. That's just exercising your eyeballs.

You don't need a memory here. Everything is done for you, living the same way day after day. Every day is a repetition of yesterday. Your caring, your meals, your routine are all done for you. You can virtually stop living.

Daisy: How do you keep up with things?

Jack: You must keep up to date with all that is newsworthy – literature, newspapers, the news. You have to go along the intelligence road. You can learn from your mistakes with your past memory. If the other residents drift down, they get depressed. Many here can't cope with the modern world, technology, etc. Even decimal currency, older people had a hell of a lot of difficulty. You have to use your intellect in the modern way of thinking for problem-solving as the older you get, the more problems you get. Depressed people can't cope with modern life.

Daisy: What's your take on dementia?

Jack: A lot of people have dementia, and they don't know they have it. They lose track of time, and they misplace things, and they don't connect it with dementia. They just think they are getting old. Many here just exist in a room, their thoughts are isolated, and they are not integrated.

Daisy: How do you manage to communicate so well with all the residents?

Jack: Sometimes you have to bring your intelligence down a few levels to communicate with them, which is unfortunate but necessary to communicate with people with mental disabilities. It's amazing how some people fall into dementia, going from an active brain to a vegetable state. Some of it is because they are not stimulated enough, no mental stimulation. It depends on what sorts of questions you ask them, and you have to listen to the answers. Give them time. Everybody has a story of their life, and you can activate their memories of bygone years. Everyone is an individual. This work is specialist work, and not many people have the interest or the intelligence to help. A lot of people here have had insular lives, and they haven't developed a life outside that.

Daisy: How do you cope seeing Bev deteriorate?

Jack: Bev doesn't extend herself to other people. We are not like man and wife now but aged friends. We've been through the good times and the bad. It's a big subject, seeing the other person going down and wondering what to do and how to help. You just become an onlooker, and other people look after her. It's a big adjustment, and there's no training for that by the way. All you have is visual contact. Even though they don't acknowledge what you are saying, they acknowledge your presence. All their visual activity is never lost. They do, though, feel your presence, which is a big support. It's a comfortable feeling. If you feel comfortable, you feel at ease, and you can relax your mind and body. If you are not comfortable, you are not receptive. Anyway, you can be thankful, when you see people deteriorating, that they have had a good life.

Daisy: How do you best ask people with dementia questions?

Jack: When you speak to these people, you have to try to jog their minds. The person you are interviewing might get brassed off, so you have to assess how much they can take as some thoughts can be very painful. The problem is the people here don't have the ability to articulate their thoughts and feelings.

Daisy: From your perspective, living here as you do, what can friends and family best do to help their loved ones here?

Jack: The thing they can do is bring information, not to just say 'nice to see you' and then just sit down and have a cup of tea. Talk about the news, what's happening. Keep you updated and informed. They need to activate your mind. Mind activation is a big thing here. They need to bring the news and get feedback from you. Ask how you are doing, how you find the meals. Are you getting a rest in the evening? Or are you dancing all night? They need to question you, not to just ask, 'How are you?' and get a yes or no answer. Ask who your friends are here. That is the best thing friends and family can do. Otherwise, people can vegetate. Nobody should vegetate.

Take them out of the environment here. Reintroduce them to the outside world, to places they went to as children. It will bring back good memories, where they used to play on the slides and swing on the swings. Take them to their favourite spots. It's all memory activation and a discussion point. Ask them if they remember being here at this spot you have taken them to. When were they here? What did they use to do? This and that. Activating their mind to the past refreshes their memories. Memories govern your life.

Daisy: Do you think it a good idea to take them to where they used to live?

Jack: Going back home involves painful memories. Then you'll start to think, 'Gosh, I lived here. I used to do this and that.'

Daisy: What's the best approach with the lower-functioning people? How do you communicate with them?

Jack: Compassion. First, you need compassion. Compassion goes a long way. And you need friendship. Don't just sit next to them and say nothing. Communicate some information to them. Eye contact is very important. It's recognition and respect. Sight and eye contact is the first thing. Greeting is the second thing, recognition and salutation, not to just come from behind and give them a fright. Remember, they may not recognise friends and family immediately, especially if they haven't seen you for a while. And also, people age. And they may have a memory of you when you were a child.

Daisy: How can relatives best help residents?

Jack: First, they have to take an interest in them. Ask the person how they are. How are they eating? How are they sleeping? Ask them what they would like to do. Would they like to go for a little drive? Go out for a coffee or an ice cream? The relatives have to go beyond themselves to the person themselves. Otherwise, it is like visiting a person in jail.

Observe their thinking capacity, their physical capacity, their emotional capacity. Capacity is needed for living. You need it for every action throughout the day. When you have the capacity to think, you then have to decide what to do with it, how to use it. You have to listen to people and give them a chance to speak. You can't disrupt them, or they will just shut up, close up, and close down.

Some think they are a cut above everyone else and look at you as though you are an idiot. People here have a lot of stories. It's important to include them and ask searching questions. Activate their minds and memory. You have to give respect. Respect is recognition, not to discourage or disparage. Some people disrupt, knocking you down. Mind wandering, I like to put it like that. The mind is wandering a bit. Losing your pattern of thinking – it's a nicer way of putting it rather than dementia.

We are all in a regimental hierarchy here. Can be soul destroying for staff and residents and the staff on the receiving end of it. You can lose your capacity to think for yourself.

Starve a person of news, and they lose their intelligence. It's as if there is nothing going on outside these four walls 'as far as they know'. Some relatives come here crowing like roosters on their perch, telling you all about them and not interested in you. Relatives can be a pain in the . . . You can see them thinking, 'I have to take time out to come and see them.'

'Christ, I wish they'd die.'

Coming in as mannequins, those who are not sure of themselves dress expensively. They go on appearances, not knowledge.

Daisy: What do the good relatives do?

Jack: Some few relatives come in and get to know the other residents and enjoy it and become a part of it. That's good.

Daisy: How do you help residents on the defensive?

Jack: Some people here are always on the defensive. They can listen and understand, but they never speak. You can't have a conversation with someone who is on the defensive. Can't have a conversation with that. They become buried in themselves, holding a resentment. They don't like being interrupted from a sleep or a lie-down. Everything becomes an imposition to the state of their living. Generally, they are people who are not sure of themselves. They have to listen, assimilate, give an answer. A lot of people can't do it anymore. Put yourself in their position. How would you feel? Some get stuck in a mindset, and some are unable to give an answer.

Daisy: What's your view of elderly carers?

Jack: A lot of relatives are aged elderly carers. They need help. They can get burnt out. They are stuffed by the time the person comes here. It's a drain on them physically and emotionally. Taxis, cars – it all costs. The aged are the carers, and the sons and daughters become the managers. They stalk around, looking at everything. The elderly carer gets really wiped out. They need rest and recuperation as well.

Grandkids are interested as family history can be passed on verbally. Grandma gives knowledge to the grandkids. Generationally, they are interested. Every ten years becomes a bygone age with the world leaping ahead so much now with technology.

Daisy: How are you finding the new residents?

Jack: We are getting a more intelligent person here now, better education, more learned of the world. They listen to the speech of the announcers and become more articulate in the way they pronounce their words. They are bringing their body and intellect into the unit.

Daisy: How do you find the staff?

Jack: The ladies here are very nice and friendly. They are not comfort ladies, but they are a comfort to have around. Better that than having big hairy, heavy-chested men making your bed. Hell! The women here are so gentle, all the laundry ladies and cleaners and carers. It's nice to have females around. They look after your needs and give comfort in the home. It is like having your mother around, quiet and gentle, comforting. They really are sweet, gentle, lovely ladies. They certainly are a gentle race, the Filipinos. The New Zealanders have a different upbringing, born to be independent.

Daisy: What problems do the residents have?

Jack: They are always trying to find the toilet, how to find their room, with their bad hips and knees. Relatives just lock them away and forget about them, saying they are in good care. Costs peace of mind sometimes. You don't even have to think about anything here. People are not used to thinking. Depends on their education and career.

Many housewives become domesticated, and they just think of their husband like a pet. They have children, look after the litter, not much to look forward to. A man can look forward to his mates, his job. He's not losing his dialogue or speech interchange with other people. Poor old Mum stuck at home with the kids in the house. Two different lifestyles under one roof, though married.

Daisy: What do you think is the best way of going about things here?

Jack: Everything has to be pieced together intelligently to make sense of it as we are doing. Then you can spoon-feed to the residents. Give a verbal test at the end to see if they have absorbed anything. At the end of the test, give a question and answer session to see what they have absorbed. Give the slower ones more time and encouragement. Give them a little test to go out and research and write it down. Better that way than just listening when it can go in the ear and out the other.

Daisy: What do you think affects the absorption rate?

Jack: Multitude of reasons – if you read, how much you read, how much you travel, how much stimulation you get, level of education, fitness level. You can go for a walk and get mental stimulation. Don't get that chance here. When you go for a walk, you can think, 'God, that's a nice car going past.' You can absorb what you are seeing and put it into your thoughts. What you see, you can recall and use in conversation. It cuts down your conversational content when you can't go out for a walk. More people should get a chance to walk outside. You can see the seasons, the gardens, the bushes, the leaves, the trees, their colours, little things of note. You can absorb what you see and gain knowledge. It's good for you physically and mentally.

Daisy: How best to help new residents?

Jack: It's a big leap in life. There is very little help around. People are thrown into this place, and they often can't cope with it. It's a complete change of life. No familiar surroundings, so they can feel lost. None of the surroundings remind you of anything, a completely different mental area for them in terms of surroundings and the people around them. To adapt to a new form of living with unfamiliar surroundings depends on your ability to adjust. We all have to integrate from all walks of life. That depends on your past life experience. If you've lived in a barracks, if you've had to problem-solve and work things out, then you can better manage here.

You have to have the ability to ask for help. You have to know how to ask the right question to get the right answer. If you ask the wrong question as a lot of people here do, you'll get the wrong answer, and that's no help. Ask the correct question to get the correct answer.

You can adjust here if you have had to adjust to a lot of different things in your life. Here, you can't cope if you've just lived in the same area where you were born, raised, went to school, married the boy down the road, had a family, and stayed in the same house. You can't then draw on those varied life experiences. They haven't had the experience of having to change to lots of different circumstances, so they get lost coming here.

Lots of people are not used to living with lots of other people and not used to speaking to lots of people. They haven't lived life in a broader sense. They have to learn to make new friends. Otherwise, they will turn into a male or female hermit.

To help them, you really have to get into their heads to understand what it is they want and try to understand what it is they are trying to ask. Some people can't express what they want. And even if they ask the right question, you are all busy and haven't time to try to explain, so they get fobbed off. It's the time factor, only twenty-four hours in the day. The people here have to wake up, think, have an opinion, and say it.

To be able to put their thoughts into words, lots of people here can't do that. They have the thoughts but not the vocabulary. They can't express themselves. They don't know how to express themselves. You have to know the person to enable them to ask the right question. People ask me questions. I don't mind. You have to get down to their level, to their mental level, to their hearing level, to their speech level, to their eye contact level. You have to recognise them as a human being.

The group is important. At least in the group, if someone says something that someone else agrees with but can't express, they can just nod and say, 'Yeah, yeah'. When they do that, you know something has sunk in. I always think, 'There but for the grace of God go I.'

8

Violence

Juliette, a big-busted, self-proclaimed sporty woman, had taken on being the defender of the vulnerable. She helped whoever needed it. The wanderers Jenny and Jonathon, who walked the corridors endlessly, had a lot less ability than the core group since they can't sit still long enough to garner any concentration. They were the odd ones out. The corridor was their home, and they circulated it up to a hundred times a day.

With little to see or entertain them on the monotonous journey, the colourful flashing TV box sitting in front of the seated group was something of a novelty as was the obstacle course of the crowded ladies' feet and their wheeled mobility walkers in front of them, walking all over the ladies' bunions, pinching their walkers, and generally getting in the way. It can work up quite a storm, especially when their favourite programmes were interrupted. Walking sticks out, the wanderers can get quite a beating.

'No, you must not do that. They are people!' Juliette shouted out.

'They don't know what they are doing.'

Resounding residents cried, 'Oh, no, they know exactly what they're doing. And they shouldn't be doing it!'

Juliette, unabashed at facing the wild denizens (having brought up three fine, upstanding sons), said, 'We are lucky to think and speak. These people can't! This is not right. This is not right. Staff, do something!'

Juliette, being the only stalwart staving off the angry crowd in this quickly escalating fight scene, was saved only by a light running staffer throwing herself unsparingly into the heap and with a few quick, non-violent karate gestures sorting it all out at lightning speed. These people deserve medals. It's dangerous stuff.

Juliette was right to defend the wanderers. If they got tipped off balance either by the intentionally placed foot, not an uncommon practice, or by other obstacles scattered about, it can mean the end of their stay at the unit. With poor balance reactions (many of them), they didn't defensively put out their arms to break their fall. So they just went down as a block, straight back, flat on their back, or crashing forwards, often head first – terrible. Quick smart, the fallen person was picked up and checked out for injuries, and if OK, they were on their way, once again looping the endless circle –hundreds and thousands of times, day in, day out. It was not an interesting track with little to see except the endless oblong cream doors, most shut tight along the way.

Daisy had witnessed it so many times, the wanderers going down. She couldn't quite believe they wouldn't bend or at least put their arm out to break their fall. She was to find out the hard way.

Taking the Friday afternoon workshop, she was up at the front, talking to the residents, when out of the corner of her eye she saw Jennifer trip over the wheel of the whiteboard. With no balance reactions, she was quickly careering to the floor. With it being near the fireplace, it was going to be a nasty fall, and Daisy couldn't bear to see her go down head first.

She seemed within reach. She was sure she could save her. She leapt backwards and, putting both arms under her armpits, cradled her. All good so far. She had caught her, thinking herself safe. But then just as quickly, Daisy felt herself careening off balance. Centre of gravity was not working this time. She was falling backwards, with Jennifer statue-like against her. Oh hell, Keith's fragile femurs were within her path, so she had to twist to avoid those.

Crash! In a split second, she was on the floor, flat on her back with Jennifer directly on top of her, expressionless and immobile. Well, that certainly didn't go as planned. How did she get that so wrong?

Staff came running. 'Are you all right?' They were genuinely concerned. It was a unique event. Staff rarely fell so dramatically.

Daisy said, 'I'm fine,' grateful to be still made of sturdy stuff, thinking, *I could have easily had a back injury out of that one.* She knew it was dangerous working here. She'd witnessed staff getting injuries and had treated quite a few, often as a physio favour at morning tea. But this was the first close call she had had herself. She'd try to be more careful in the future.

*   *   *

Gabrielle had been at the unit for four years. She knew all the ropes and certainly pulled them, all to her own advantage. Short and built like a barrel with a bark on her that would scare any dog, few can stand up to her.

She hated showering. It took three Filipino staff (best if one was a male) to shower her, shouting match all the way. Her visceral screaming can be heard right through to the reception lobby. Where did that woman get such vocal strength? Definitely not good PR for visitors. Those screams really reverberated.

Plenty of war wounds came out of it, really bad-looking big welts. The generally modest staff flaunted their battle bruises bravely at breaks like the tough little cookies that they were. Their battle team tactics were phenomenal. All their Filipino finesse of gracefully swift-moving arms and legs at forty-five kilos of body weight or less was a sight to behold.

Not so with Daisy. She found Gabrielle scary with her bull-rushing tactics on both staff and residents, karate kicking and body throwing. Definitely not for her. She had to find another way.

To the rescue was Jack Reacher. She was binge-reading Lee Child. Reacher became a real confidant. He explained in fight scenes that you had to 'get close so they can't land a punch. Stand tall, full size. Chest out and face them full on.' This all sounded very confronting to Daisy, but still, she had to try something.

Daisy was no weakling. She'd faced many a tough resident in her time but nothing like this. Gabrielle was full-on formidable. Anyway, what must be done must be done.

So mustering up the courage and putting Juliette to her right as a handy sidekick and Jack Reacher as left hemisphere arsenal, Daisy launched forth. David and Goliath. With Gabrielle rushing forth, shouting, and spitting, Daisy mustered up her full height, a handy five feet ten inches, and towering over her applied the 'get close, chest out' commandeering profile. Gabrielle faltered and, crumpling like Christmas paper, acquiesced. Amazing. Jack Reacher had worked. There was no trouble since for Daisy.

Not daunted in her tracks, though, Gabrielle still preyed on and intimidated new residents, especially in their first few weeks of coming to the unit, at their most vulnerable. She was pestering and provoking them before they'd had a chance to make new friends and garner a measure of support. For the frailer, more timid ladies, it was terrifying.

Gabrielle squatted at the coveted two-bay window seat, pushing off unsuspecting contenders, aiming for the second vacant seat, giving an extra shove for good measure, saying, 'It's mine!' She was plummeting the unit's falls rating and worse still if the victim got a broken femur out of it.

Juliette, with her strong sense of justice and sporty feistiness of 'I'm sporty, and I'm strong', was the only one who had the guts to stand up to her. Courageous and having size and weight on her side, she regularly called out for staff recruits, 'This is not right. This is not right! You have to do something!' all while Gabrielle was violating. Though Juliette was right, staff had a hard enough time attending to their ever-burgeoning work schedules without breaking up fights as well. They can't be in two places at once, though many would demand them be.

Daisy took Jack Reacher to the unit, *Worth Dying For.* Reading an extract to them, they were all enthralled. It was an instant hit. They loved him.

Theodora said Lee Child was her son's favourite author, and she just had to have that very copy there and then. Always keen to support literary ventures, Daisy relinquished it with some regret as it was her favourite cover, the expensive version. You could see Jack Reacher either surveying the barren, burnt Nebraska country from the cliff back to you or just as easily coming down the embankment, all shoulders and thighs your way. Theodora promptly snatched the book, coveted cover now gone and now sitting pride of place on her much-worn walker seat. The rest of the series, twenty-one books, Daisy had borrowed from a friend, all printed in Vietnam. Cheaper, yes, but Reacher's frame on the cover had shrunk by about 40 per cent. Not quite the same.

Theodora was the only resident who had managed to build up a floor library in her room – high piles of earmarked books, half-completed crossword puzzles, the women's magazines her daughter brought, and special articles from the *Saturday Press*. These teetering renditions were balanced tentatively all round her walls. Such ramshackle sights would be whisked away in other rooms, but she somehow managed to restrain staff from removing them. Always reading something, she was never without a book or magazine in her hand. She certainly knew how to maximise her walking seat, regularly putting the equivalent of four magazines, three books, one big full cup of tea, a piece of cake, and a pile of rescue tissues on top.

If the tea spilled, which it often did, she said, 'Oh, just mop it up with these tissues.' They were never enough. So she was off again to the kitchen to get yet more paper towels. She totally expected this hands-on service. She was paying for it, wasn't she? As she said proudly, she came from a wealthy family, and money had never been a problem. Her father owned a factory and used to make uniforms for the soldiers in the war, so with that revenue, all the eleven children fared quite well.

'Just do your job and be done with it,' she'd say as you were quickly mopping up what was spilt. Wouldn't like to be employed in her household! No doubt she'd employed staff, but you'd have to wonder how long they stayed.

*   *   *

There were only four double bay windows, all set facing the sun and overlooking the award-winning garden where you got to see the visitors coming and going. If you were lucky enough, you might get to spy a lovely little child jumping up and down or a tiny fluffy dog straining at a lead, plenty of them. For these captivating reasons, it was understandable that window seats were highly sought after.

So there were eight window seats, minus two as Gabrielle's guarding those, leaving only six seats for twenty-eight residents. Juliette had the privilege of sitting next to her, the only one with this dubious honour. Comrade in arms so to speak. Gabrielle had met her match.

Complaining bitterly that it was unfair for the others, Juliette, nevertheless, still let her sit there. She was not stupid enough to sacrifice a window seat in the sun when there was a chance for it. They were hard enough to get as it was. Such were the days at the dementia unit, pecking order all the way and a tough place to make your way in.

'Why is that Gabrielle woman still there?' you may well ask. 'Shouldn't she be shipped off to some other place?' One would think so, but Rome wasn't built in a day, and things can move mysteriously slowly in such places. Other things can be frighteningly fast, like when you see bodies shipped out the door with only a thin white sheet covering them, in hushed tones, without anyone saying a word. You can see the hearse taking it away, but no one is told who it is or where it came from, and you don't very much feel like asking.

Daisy couldn't work out how Gabrielle was getting away with all this aggressive behaviour either. Then one fine Friday morning, she discovered how. Gabrielle's handsome tall doctor arrived to see her. On entry, she immediately metamorphosed. Putting on a maiden's wanton gaze and smiling benignly, she fluttered long-gone eyelashes while clasping her hands to an enlarged waist, like Falstaff, and simpering. It beggared belief to witness it. You would think it fiction if you weren't actually seeing it for yourself.

The staging worked perfectly for her. How could anyone imagine her otherwise? She had been at the unit for four good long years with no sign of leaving and still strong as an ox, so things weren't likely to change in a hurry.

While visitors were often helpful and afforded a limited measure of safety, it was the 24/7 threat that residents needed to be protected from. Staff did what they can, but the best help was often from one another. Juliette was exceptional. She protected everyone. But mostly, it was your friends who stuck up for you. Oh yes, and Jack, he'd protect the ladies if the male residents were having a go. But that often ended up in a fight, which didn't help anybody either.

Your friend was your greatest ally. Anyone can get out their walking stick and yell out for you, if they had to. And they did.

About half the residents at the unit had the capacity to be violent or do harm if they wanted to, and less than half of that group again exerted that ability at some point and to varying degrees. Some were more actively aggressive than others, Gabrielle being an extreme case in terms of constancy and dominance.

Then there were those who were naturally nice and sweet. They went up behind the ladies and tickled them gently on the back of their neck. For those in high-alert vigilance, getting that instead of an imagined thump on the head was disconcerting at best. It was hard to know whether to laugh in relief or scream out in frustration.

It was important not to overlook the wanderers. Residents had a lot to contend with day in, day out, especially the wanderers. It was a long day for them, roaming the corridors, only really sitting at mealtimes.

Ron was one of the unit's long-term residents and a wanderer. Only in his sixties, he was well cared for by staff and family. It had reached the point where his mobility was seizing up, and he had to be transferred to the hospital.

Daisy was sitting at the desk when Ron's daughters came in with chocolates and a card to thank the staff. Daisy said, 'I'll get the charge nurse.' On most occasions, Daisy was told not to talk to relatives.

The daughters quickly interjected, 'No, we're happy to talk to you.'

They said how much they appreciated the care and concern for their father, saying, 'He was the least stressed he'd ever been. All his life, he'd been super busy with his painting business.' They were now pleased to see him chilled and happy. Daisy listened, encouraged.

They had learnt to communicate with Ron without the traditional verbal communication. He had dementia when he was younger, and often then, people are hit harder with the disease, and speech goes rapidly, many becoming wanderers, and their ability to learn and engage becomes a lot more difficult than when onset is in an older person. As regular visitors, the daughters had no resentment, always upbeat. His happiness was their primary concern. *Selfless*, Daisy thought, *inspiring*.

Jennifer, the other wanderer who had just fallen on top of Daisy the previous week, came up to her. Patting her on the head as she would have a pony, she said clear as a bell, 'You are lovely.'

Seizing the opportunity (as she rarely spoke), Daisy said, 'Jennifer, you need to be alert where you walk. Last week, you fell over the whiteboard wheel, and I tried to catch you, and we both fell, you on top of me.

'Oh dear', she said.

'You have to be very careful,' Daisy said.

She replied with a remorseful yes.

She is so lovely, Daisy thought, *with hardly any warmth of human contact.* She had loved animals, breeding show ponies, and had won many awards. You could see how animals would have responded to her kindness. And you could see from the pictures on her walls that they did.

Jenny loved dancing in a palm tree sort of way. Still, there was no trunk rotation, but her body-waving style was starting to attract interest. Other residents were now getting the confidence to try their style on the increasingly full dance floor mid-exercise class before an absolute no-no as 'There could be falls!' For now, the staff turned a blind eye.

In her element, dancing, the charge nurse could see Jenny smiling. 'Happy Jennifer?'

'Yes', came the reply.

9

Community

'I love everybody,' said Juliette, answering Daisy's question of How do you help new residents coming into the unit? 'I just say, "Hello. I've just come to say hello to you and ask, 'How are you?'" I don't just go in and say, "It is lovely," because it takes time to adjust. I say, "We are happy having you here. We are happy you are here as there are a lot of people here of our age. We are well looked after. The meals are nice. That's important. I explain to them that they will like this place, that we are well looked after, that the staff are lovely, and we have to be happy. No grumpy here. If you are eating everything you like, you are happy. No cooking here. We don't have to work, just enjoy it. And we have a few men here, and it is good. It's nice to have a few men with us.'

That was the longest monologue Juliette had given certainly that Daisy had witnessed. To date, it had just been her standard auto-repeat lines of 'We are getting old,' 'We must be positive,' 'We mustn't get grumpy,' and of course 'Staff, do something!'

'Congratulations, Juliette,' Daisy said. 'You are really stretching your thinking. You are thinking really well.'

Juliette beamed her accomplished netballer look.

Daisy was about to ask others when there was a nearby shriek that would make anybody's blood curdle. 'Do something. She has been like that all day. She has nearly driven me mad!'

Jack went over and said, 'It's OK, Nan. She is my wife. So she is OK. I can see her from over here.'

'Sorry, I have to tell you, but she has been sitting here doing nothing at all. She has been doing this all day, nothing. Move her. She is driving me mad!'

Jack, losing his patience, was about to take a lunge when nurses quickly scuttled in. 'She is just sleeping,' they said. They said sorry to Jack and quickly manoeuvred Beverly out of the way; things settled down.

Nan never slept in public and conscientiously folded tea towels all day long. If others didn't do similar, they were ignorant loafers as far as she was concerned.

At this rate, Daisy was lucky to get a good run of ten minutes or more without a feigned or real emergency breaking out. *It's amazing,* she thought, *that the residents aren't in a worse state in such a highly adrenalised environment.*

With Nancy's scream, David alighted upon the opportunity to change into the newly acquired role of guru master, picked up from who knows where as Suzy said he'd never done yoga before. With outstretched arms and now lotus-looking fingers, he said, 'Now follow me, everyone. Breathe. After me. Breathe in . . . and breathe out. In . . . and out. Calm down . . . just calmly now . . . gently. Lovely, just like me.'

Daisy took the advice. Then they were back to the topic of helping new residents.

Patsy, a new resident herself, had adjusted remarkably well. Sense of humour helped, and she had a good one. She had made friends readily and said, 'Everything's super. I haven't really had to adjust. Everyone is nice and friendly. I mean that too. I'm not being silly. It is a lovely place. How can we be grumpy? We have a good outlook. Look out the window. It's a beautiful scene outside. Quite a change coming into here. It's doing something different. When you come through the door and look around, you can see that it is a big place. Quite a change to your ordinary home or house. It's not what you have been doing. It really isn't. Look around. It's really lovely.'

What an incredible person, Daisy thought. No complaints. She knew she had a spartan room. She'd just seen it. There was nothing in it. Not even a comfortable chair had been brought in. It was no better than a hospital ward. But still, here she was, espousing good will and tolerance.

That was why she liked working here. Many residents were living in stark abstemious conditions with no resources from outside. A monastery would have appeared lavish compared with many of their rooms. Still, often with just a few clothes hanging in the wardrobe, uncomplainingly, they have the grace to rise above it all. She admired the way this generation never complained. Never speaking ill of their children, no matter what support was or wasn't given, they stoically carried on regardless.

'You have to adjust to the place, the people, and the lifestyle,' said Jack. 'It's a fact of life, giving up property. People are born, live, get old, and become sedentary. A big part of it is how you have lived. If you had a gratifying life, it's a successful life. When you look around, you can almost feel the memory bank, thousands of years of history here. Your outlook is what helps you adjust. It's amazing how integration happens, just listening to the people, like a pair of knitting needles just knitting everything together. Amazing how it all works out. It takes time to get to know each other. We are in a big community of old people, and everyone is adapting. It is a big learning curve for everyone. Life is a learning curve. Being old is still a learning curve – how to interact with one another, how to think. What you can't do, just forget about it. Find something new. Nothing should annoy you here. Don't let it fester. Otherwise, it is very distressing, in fact. It can grow out of all proportion. People need to settle down. Sort out the problem. If you don't settle down, you can't sort out the problem.'

It's true about the learning curve, thought Daisy. Jack was certainly flourishing in the group.

'I look around my room, and I might need this or that for a little bit of a change because it is my home,' said the newly confident Juliette.

'Memorabilia', said Jack. 'You see the picture, and it takes you back. You remember who you are.'

David, meanwhile, had unfurled himself out of his coiled, meditative position and with accrued confidence stood and took the floor. He'd done a lot of public speaking for his coastal patrol work and won awards for it, so he felt he could do the same now. He had a strong voice and could speak to a crowd with ease. So standing tall, he announced, 'Look, we have a team of people. People have to learn to teach their own. If you have made a mistake, talk about it. And all of a sudden, you have achieved. Smile at yourselves. Attract positive about you. Smooth it all away. If you have a fight, talk about it and become friends. We are all trying to adjust. Now I want you to do an exercise. All stand up and point your arm out straight with your finger pointed and turn a full 360 degrees.'

Stony silence. No one moved, standing up being an effort for many. Daisy, though, obliged. She stood up and, pointing her finger at the end of her outstretched arm, turned the full circle.

'Now all the people you have pointed to, ask yourself the question Have you respect for them? If you have, we will win,' said David.

'An excellent exercise', Daisy said to the group. 'We can all learn from that. Thank you, David.'

Jack was paying attention to David, but Theodora, usually the centre of attention, was getting fed up. Shoving Jack in the ribs, she said, 'How are you finding this? What's he going on about? We don't want to listen to this. It's a waste of time, nothing new, not learning anything.'

To Jack's credit, he said nothing and remained neutral. Theodora promptly moved. It was the first time ever that she hadn't managed to disrupt the group or get a rise when she wanted to. Articulate, she usually could; but overpowered this time, she walked off to more conciliatory pastures.

'You have to invite and include but not force. Don't push others. Shouldn't be an imposition. Don't push people into a corner,' said Doreen from the corner, a well-dressed tiny woman with wild grey hair who often dressed in very bright pink. Daisy wasn't sure what she meant. Maybe she was referring to her. She should have asked but missed the opportunity.

Either way, it was good for David to speak out as he didn't usually speak out in the group. This was his first time. Usually, it was Theodora and Jack who took the floor.

Theodora would come back. She had confidence and the solace of her magazines. She knew everything in them. She'd just corrected Daisy on Boris Johnson going to Cambridge. 'He went to Oxford, didn't he?'

David sat down. He was always saying, 'I want to help,' and didn't seem to be getting anywhere with his repeated requests. Having been in the police force, he had plenty of wide-ranging experiences. He knew he could help, and he wanted to. He decided to start things up himself. His first initiative was sitting with the unwell residents. He'd sit for hours, holding the hands of the sick and the often dying.

Staff, realising he had a gift for it, started wheeling up the seriously unwell person on the mobile recliner to be with him. He said he was there to 'be there and listen'. He was very compassionate and never got angry, frustrated, or upset. If a woman, he was sensitive enough to know whether to hold her hand. If a man, he'd just place his hand gently on top. Especially for those people who didn't get visitors, even at such a time, it was a great social service.

Everybody had somebody. But they didn't always visit. Unmarried immigrants were the least likely to have visitors. One such was Isabella, a British immigrant, once a university geography lecturer. Her POA was a former student. She came in with her partner saying enthusiastically that they would be visiting more often as they'd just moved into a house nearby. Daisy was sure they would, judging by her enthusiasm.

'We'll see,' said Isabella reservedly. Unfortunately, they didn't come or at least not while Daisy was working.

Isabella was of similar persona to Janet in way of institutionalised academia, Isabella with geography, Janet in accounting. But at least Janet joined in with the group where much was received from both sides of the equation. But Isabella could never bring herself to do that. She'd listen but never contribute. She could have, having a pile of filled-in crosswords by her chair to prove it.

You could see she'd devoted herself to her work with all her framed certificates on the walls. She'd obviously had an esteemed career, but it was tough at the end when there were neither friends or family at your side, away from your own country where you were more likely to have them. Daisy and others made an effort to bridge the gap, but none had ever been able to.

Daisy noticed on reflection that it was former university lecturers and high school teachers who tended to be like this, distant and less likely to join in, but not nurses or primary school teachers. They were full participants. Or all had been to date. Interesting. She hadn't noticed till now. She wondered how ex-physiotherapists fared.

David was near suicidal when he came in. Now with his new-found sense of purpose with comforting the sick, he'd found meaning. It had lifted his spirits remarkably. Previously morose and depressed, he was now bounced back with a spring in his step and a renewed sense of humour.

He was so amenable that staff had taken the unusual step of taking him from the higher functioning table where his neighbour Nell was to the tough table, supposedly downgrading if you like. At his dining table of four, he had Gabrielle to his left; the blind man, Ivan, who needed lots of support, on his right; and Jenny, the wanderer who spoke little, on the far side. Comfortable and thinking nothing of it, David wouldn't think of moving. Who else would sit next to Gabrielle with her irrational, violating ways? No one, not with the way she lashed out and insulted, often without a trigger so you'd never know when it was coming.

David was unperturbed. Being a former detective, and a strong man at that, he considered it all nothing out of the ordinary. Not intimidated, he ate his meal beside her without an ounce of tension, unlike the other ladies at Nell's table behind, squirming at the look of her and wondering when the next plate would go flying.

Nell was a friend of David and the best turnout woman in the unit. She had streaked hair with good-quality haircuts and was still with her own hairdresser. All her Lancôme make-up was lined up on her dresser, Chanel perfume in the bathroom, and cashmere cardigans and good suede shoes in the wardrobe. How she kept it all out of the way of pilfering wanderers Daisy had no idea. The family must bring in refills without comment as you never heard complaints.

Though personable and pleasant, Nell had always kept her distance. David was the only one she befriended. She was well aware of his problem with Marina. Seeing him locked up in the nurses' station doing jigsaw puzzles just to get away from her wasn't right as far as she was concerned.

Daisy went to meet her in her room to see if they could work out a plan to help. She couldn't have been nicer, ushering her into the best room on the floor, with her cream leather lounger facing a good garden view and self-embroidered pictures above it. Fragrance sticks sent out welcoming aromas, and amidst them, Daisy and Nell talked.

'Yes, David's a great guy,' she said. 'I'm a friend of the family, and Suzy takes me out with them sometimes. That Marina who goes after David is terrible though. Can't something be done? Otherwise, the rest of the patients are all very good. I like to help him if I can.'

They discussed further and came up with a David protection scheme. Both Daisy and Nell would keep on the lookout, and if Marina came anywhere near him, they would sound the alarm and shoo her off. Nell had a strong voice and could use it ably, as could many of the women on the floor, so he had a strong and capable ally.

It only seemed to take a few well-timed interventions, and within a week, Marina was out of the way. It was seemingly too difficult to make her way in. The neighbourhood watch at work had stifled her. *Remarkable result*, Daisy thought. She wasn't sure she wouldn't re-emerge though. Sphinx from the ashes so to speak. But still, for now, she was submerged. It was success enough in itself. David was now free to go back to his hospice work.

Daisy was impressed with how committed residents were to helping one another. *Could teach us a thing or two*, she thought. And it wasn't just about residents helping residents anymore. Sometimes it was residents helping staff.

Daisy was in Jack's room, asking a few questions, when one of the cleaners came in. She had the loveliest smile, as they all did, and was just a wisp of a thing. Here she was, carrying around yet another monstrous piece of equipment, almost triple her size, a groaning, lopsided laundry trolley. It was amazing she could even manoeuvre it.

Looking closer, Daisy could see she was not from the Philippines, as most staff were, with those big doll-like eyes. Asking further, she found out she was Korean. 'Korean', Jack promptly said. 'I was on active service in the Korean War from 1950 to 1953.'

She was overjoyed to have someone who understood her homeland amidst a workforce who hardly knew one.

Daisy left. She knew Jack would have some special stories for her. She was happy that this lovely girl was going to get some hard-earned history from her homeland she probably didn't even know herself. With Jack having such good recall, Daisy knew she was going to get some valuable insights and information.

When next meeting in the kitchen, the Korean girl said, 'You wouldn't know he had dementia. He has such a good memory.' He had explained the incredible hardships the North Korean people went through, coming south through a war zone with their families, just what they had on their backs, then the hardship of building a life from scratch, literally with nothing. She said a lot of this history was lost to her generation as no one discussed it with them. She was incredibly happy to have been able to do so with Jack.

What touched her most was the sweets and the chocolates, how the soldiers carried them around in their pockets and would give them out to all the Korean children. That would be Jack. All the world around. it's the heartfelt gestures that are remembered the most.

10

Departure

Jane's son was visiting. He noticed Shirlene's daughter Jolene and thought, *An interesting woman. I'd like to meet her.* So with usual due diligence, he did and discovered she was, yes, a model (few who looked like her weren't) and that, yes, she had actually set up the first modelling and fashion agency for girls in the Middle East.

Now that was something, he thought. *You don't meet that every day.* Enquiring further, one for drilling deep, he discovered that, yes, she did still have the glamorous beaded gowns, and would she model them? Well, yes, she could, and would she? Well, yes, she would.

So that was confirmed. It was a mega-celebrity event. Everyone was invited. And of course, they came – the catwalk, the drinks and nibbles, the works. The special care fashion show on 5 April was a celebrity event. Relatives all arrived this time. That was for sure, not wanting to miss the rarefied glitz and glamour.

It may have seemed otherwise, but the residents came first in David and Jolene's eyes. Both were extremely good to their parents with a real concern and interest in helping and uplifting the residents as well. Remember the caring relative who left a note on her mother's heater when the rooms were near to deep frozen? That was Jolene, a glamorous tall model who was devoted to her mother and spent hours each day attending to her.

Shirlene had had a pampered life – three husbands, plenty of Mediterranean cruises, and a luxuriating life which her tsarina looks well afforded. A lovely woman and perfectly charming, she relied on her daughter (probably overly) as she did on her husbands prior.

Shirlene's pampering schedule was noteworthy. First thing was the make-up. Jolene came in daily, beauty kit in hand (one in the bedroom, a spare in the handbag), and set about doing the elaborate make-up and hair routine. Everything was at work – teasing, perfuming, painting, polishing. It was not for the faint-hearted, especially if done daily as Shirlene's was. No wonder at 95, she still looked resplendent. It was labour-intensive business, no doubt expensive as well.

Most residents hardly had this sort of manicure on their wedding day, let alone as a daily routine. Awestruck, they watched on in unholy envy. Unaware of onlookers, Jolene performed with due diligence – teased the curls (*Why did those girls wash Mum's hair when she had just had it set? No need!*); adjusted the jewellery, of which there were many a set; and set the mohair blanket just right and there. That was it. Nothing less would do. Shirlene came out looking splendid from these revitalising beauty rituals, emerging polite and pleasant but imperious nevertheless. Relying on her daughter far too much, Shirlene was aware of it. Still, she didn't really want to go to the effort of making new friends when she had her daughter's attention and regular morning rites to look forward to.

Preparations were underway for the big day. It finally arrived. Everyone dressed in their best clothes, hair combed, lipstick on for those who had it, red carpet laid out. Staff were busy laying out all the tasty hors d'oeuvre specially put together in the kitchen. Residents and relatives were on either side of the catwalk. The place was transformed to a celebrity fashion show. There was one in a million chance of this happening here.

The glorious, glamorous sequinned gowns were something out of a fairy tale, not exactly putting Lady Di to shame but certainly challenging her. How could someone look like that in their seventies? (Think Joanna Lumley.) Jolene graced the catwalk in superstar splendour. Thirty glorious gowns were paraded down the central aisle with daring allure and all with exquisitely purpose-made jewels for each ensemble. And the stylised stiletto heels, on those points for a whole afternoon! Never a waver, a pure professional.

All the traditional Arab dress was modelled, the abaya, a simple long black maxi dress with the hijab headscarf, and then the face cover with the burka. You could only see the eyes through a very small slit or an attractively enmeshed enclave. What if they needed glasses? That would make it doubly difficult. Ominous and unnerving, exotic and eclectic, hard to know which. Such an extreme duality from what they were wearing beneath.

Daisy wondered how these women survive back in their countries. Dressed like this in such hot weather, often in black, it must have been like a sauna.

The men at least had long loose white robes which reflected the sun at least rather than absorbed it as black goes. Then there was the royal-looking turban headgear, in the Middle East at least. Their faces were showing, and everything was gleaming white. Of course, they were going to make a better show of it than the funereal-looking women.

Then it was breakout time, outer black discarded. It was mostly Western gowns that were worn for weddings, lots of bright colours, gold jewellery, and shimmer. Such gowns Jolene was modelling, royalty Middle East style.

Daisy had never witnessed anything like it and in all likelihood neither had her compatriots. This apparel was for the super elite, nothing spared, usually witnessed from afar. To see them so close up with all the gloss and sheen, fabrics, mosaics, patterns, colours, and allure was spellbinding. What a treat. What a new-found privilege. Residents could hardly believe what they were seeing.

Jolene had brought all these beautifully bejewelled gowns from Dubai, all packed and labelled. Looking as if brand new from the box, just off the rack, they were breathtaking. You could hardly imagine it being topped, Chanel and Karl Lagerfeld's creations notwithstanding.

Residents couldn't help but be awestruck by the performance, utterly mesmerising. Jane and Shirlene were front row in special seats, loving every minute, Shirlene for the glamour and Jane sitting next to David saying, 'I feel myself coming back.' Relatives couldn't resist it. The throngs were pushing right to the front line. Residents were almost pushed onto the catwalk.

The Filipino staff quickly outmanoeuvred everyone, handing out the drinks and plentiful exotic savouries. This was something indeed. Anyone would be hard-pressed to find an event like this in town or indeed in the country for that matter.

David – strong, sporty, and statuesque – worked the crowd, entertaining the enthralled relatives, now guests. The show turned out to be stunningly spectacular. It went off without a hitch. He and Jolene had pulled off quite a feat, Jolene having done most of the work. But David's encouragement made it happen. It could have been on any cover of any magazine, *Vogue* included.

The spectacular experience stayed with the residents for weeks. They both recognised and appreciated the efforts that had been made for them, thanking Jolene, saying, 'Thank you for doing this for our entertainment.'

Really, thought Daisy, *photos should have been taken to be used to promote the residents and the unit in a more positive light.* But Privacy Act was strongly in place. Easier said than done.

Anyway, first, the residents had to be given the chance to thrive and excel. This event had certainly done that. The message had to get out somehow, what the residents were achieving. They needed someone to champion them, much like Sir John Kirwan had done for depression. He had certainly changed the face of it, a New Zealand icon admitting the problem, and all of a sudden, it was normalised. Everyone was talking about it, stigma practically gone. That needed to happen for dementia. Alzheimer's New Zealand had champions speaking on dementia. That was a good start, ably speaking on creating networks and getting help and how creative ways of communicating needed to be developed.

That weekend, Jane went up to North Canterbury to stay on the farm with David, always coming back refreshed and invigorated. Going every few months, she loved it, being outdoors, everything that was familiar to her. Few residents went out overnight. And with the long car trip there and back, it was a testament to her strength and David's consideration that such weekends went ahead.

Then disaster struck. David mysteriously had to leave the country. He never really told Jane why – that she could recall anyway. Jane was devastated. Nothing could console her. She never recovered. Not one to cry or show her emotions, she buried them stoically. All she would say was, 'A good man's gone.'

If Daisy ever bought him up, she'd say, 'I don't want to talk about it!' He was as good as dead in her eyes. All emotions were turned inwards, festering and brewing. Soon they'd erupt.

After his departure, Jane's family decided to cut Daisy's work, citing that help was no longer needed. This decision cut both Jane's life lines. She was now rudderless.

Daisy went to see her after the redundancy, and Jane said, 'I don't want to sit up. I think they are wanting to take you off me.' Daisy went to see her on Friday nights after work; it was never quite the same.

Jane knew she'd been abandoned and said, 'They have stopped us playing. I can't do it. I need your help.'

Soon after, Jane's anger exploded, now with no training, no David, no Daisy, no support in place for her. She couldn't control her 'fuzzy mind, fuzzy brain'. So it just took over. Wildly, she'd lash out at staff and residents, whoever got in the way, usually saying, 'They don't understand.' She didn't have David's persuasive phone calls anymore and no Daisy to make them. She had no chance to try anymore.

Jane had liked the discipline of the training, and Daisy had become a good friend. Now with all that taken away, there was no support or structure for her to hold on to. Anger blinded. She even started becoming aggressive towards Angela, who'd been looking after Jane for more than six years. It was then that Daisy realised the seriousness. To lash out at her last support proved she'd lost all control.

Losing her appetite, she plummeted to less than forty-five kilograms in dramatic fashion. Angela tried to get her to eat but with little success. Even the protein drink wasn't building her up. All efforts seemed to be to no avail. Now so thin, it was shocking to witness.

Still, miraculously, she maintained a formidable strength. She hit out at carers with ever-increasing violence; they now sported eye-watering welts and mottled brown bruises all over their arms. Staff were brought to tears.

Going into Jane's room, Daisy explained to her what she'd done. Initially, she denied it, saying, 'You're lying. I didn't do it.'

Daisy had Angela come in and show Jane the bruising injury. Jane, embarrassed and repentant, said 'I'm sorry' repeatedly with various shades of remorse. Daisy asked her, 'Do you want me to keep telling you when you're hitting out at people?'

Jane said, 'You have to tell me. I have to know.'

But without the support and the accrued discipline from her training, Jane lost all tolerance and restraint, and the attacks increased. Daisy found it terrible witnessing the injuries and also seeing what was happening to Jane. She was now wrist-burning the residents and had a formidable grip that took two to untangle.

Daisy was a recipient of one such attack in the lounge. Foolishly thinking it would be different for her, she bent down to talk to Jane, hoping to establish eye contact. No such luck. Without recognition and as quick as a whip, Jane came out with one powerful punch to her stomach and then a lightning strike to her jaw, straight to the top set of teeth, frighteningly quick. Daisy hardly had time to register, her first concern being, *This could be one very expensive dental bill!*

Trying to stop her, Daisy went to grab Jane's wrist, but she grabbed hers faster and then started twisting it. This little, forty-four-kilogram woman, how was this even possible? It was getting tighter and tighter, and Daisy was sure she could release her grip if she could just get in there and apply the right amount of force. Her strength had never failed her before, and she didn't want this to be the moment that it did! Still, the pain was ratcheting up.

Eventually, she was forced to call out. It was too painful. The grip was unyielding. Help, though, was not fast in coming. Having been through this before but seemingly not on himself, the good nurse sauntered over, not breaking stride, all this after Daisy's second plaintive call. Being a big man, he released her.

Attacks were now happening daily and often multiple times. There was not always a male staffer around, no policy for that. Daisy was just lucky that one was there when she needed the help, albeit slow in coming. With so many attacks, it was becoming more and more difficult to record them all. Fast and furious, it was becoming a tidal wave.

On a Friday night, Daisy would still go and watch the Southern Alps sunset with her. The friendship was still here. You could feel it. But the 'fuzzy brain fuzzy mind' had definitely taken over.

Daisy felt that when Jane attacked her, she wasn't seeing her, not just no recognition. She was seeing something else. Her eyes had a glazed, wild look with no semblance of the old Jane Daisy once knew.

On arriving at work the next week, Jane wasn't there. She'd been sent onto a higher level of dementia care. There, they had authority to restrain you for attacking staff or other residents. Apparently, her daughters came in to pack up the room.

So that was it. The 'racing mind, fuzzy brain' pioneer had gone with all that good work, all her effort and interest and trying, all her conscious goodwill for others, all her broad thinking and big plans. She couldn't just go like that. What about her legacy? What about all the others who needed the help?

It seemed so unusually quiet. Daisy was distraught. David and Jane were both gone, the two pillars in the work. What now?

Jane had always known the programme wasn't just for her. It was a pioneering work not just for those in the unit but also for others beyond. She was inspired by the fact that the work was helping others. Through her enormous efforts and explanations, Daisy had been better able to understand the dementia experience and 'fuzzy brain' and 'fuzzy mind' and progress the work forward.

11

Positivity

'Dad just said Granny's been admitted to the unit, so I came straight here,' she told Daisy. This ingenious girl somehow managed to bypass the 'wait one week till your relative settles in' regime. Still, though, that night, disorientated and lonely, her dear granny Win became very upset. With the family informed, the four arrived in tour de force the next morning, setting themselves up on the veranda outside.

Win was now wrapped in a rug and large woolly jumper to fend off the chilly, autumnal air, holding a large steaming cup of coffee that her granddaughter, bypassing kitchen protocol, had just made. The son brought out his weighty guitar and started strumming all his mother's favourites with a familiar reach and a well-tuned, articulate tension. His magnificent voice soared through the doors and ceilings. *What a beautiful welcome*, Daisy thought.

The family of four then descended for lunch, cramming themselves into Win's already congested table. The granddaughter was a real natural with the elderly and quickly made friends with everyone. Introducing herself as Win's granddaughter, she quickly garnered names from everyone. The residents quickly fell in love with her and, by association, Win.

Now saved from all that awkwardness of having to meet new people, Win was visibly relieved. She found that sort of thing difficult, given her shyness, age, and failing memory. Juliette, being at Win's table, was pleased to show off her new-found elocution skills. She praised the place and everyone in it. Win was welcomed in.

Her son realised pretty quickly that if his mother could make friends from the start, her quality of life would improve markedly. Any way they could help, they would do it. They all stayed for Win's extended lunch, choosing not to have anything themselves. If they had, they'd have been whisked away to another table and not had any chance to get to know Win's compatriots. Bypassing etiquette again, they just squashed themselves in. Juliette's table had never had such fun, just like Christmas Day. Staff weren't quite sure how to handle this self-starter group of troubadour relatives not having developed a skill set for such.

About to go, the son could see Win was getting anxious. So reassuring and drawing her over, he said, 'Come over here, Mum, and we'll give you a good hug. You've had lots of music and a good chat with the other folk at lunch. So you have good company when we are not here. See you very soon, Mum.'

Daisy was doing her notes at the prescribed exit and couldn't help but say under her breath, 'That's the best farewell I've seen.' The son heard and tried not to do a double take. Inappropriate maybe, but she'd viewed thousands, so she felt it warranted comment.

Undeterred he said, 'OK, Mum, one more hug.'

'Bye, Gran,' said the granddaughter and yet another.

Glory days, Daisy thought. *Let's hope we get more of these.*

Win had just told her, 'Family is the most important.' Daisy had just witnessed now how.

Beaming, Win now had new friends and all introduced by her very own family – no abandonment, no sudden isolation, complete and total support, the best way to integrate by far. The majority aren't that fortunate, though, to have such a family that will welcome them in as Win's just had. So if not, take Jack's approach.

His three sons hadn't visited for an age, and whilst it had broken his wife's spirit, Jack had determined that it wouldn't his. 'Don't need a family as we've one here. This is the family now. We live here. Room is here. Have meals here, conversations and company here, all the comforts of home. Family's just expanded,' he said explicitly.

'You just have to change your lifestyle, eating habits, mealtimes, routine. Being in the same lounge with other people instead of in your own lounge, you need to be able to converse with others.'

Residents were starting to open up. There was a lot more discussion going on, not just from Theodora and Jack. Juliette, David, and Patsy had started to increase their dialogue as well. Jack was now sitting in the front row rather than the back stalls as prior. With him now contributing more to the group, even Theodora was curbing her imperious ways to accommodate Jack's more magnanimous ones.

This was outlined in an interesting turn of events at the Saturday afternoon karaoke session. Golden oldies but goodies were playing. Singing along to 'You Are My Destiny', a big number and one of the favourites, Jack remarked, 'It's amazing that they can come up with all these words and match the music to it.' It looked to be the first time he'd considered it. And maybe it was. He seemed all the more potent with the ever-attentive Theodora alluringly at his side, awkward but somehow working.

Marina now having faded, fortunate as he couldn't discuss anything with her, Theodora had risen in not just confidence but also humility now it seemed, so much so that during one such serenade, she must have had a memory lapse. She turned to Jack and said, 'Who are you?'

With good humour, he replied, 'Jack.'

'Oh, yes, of course.'

Not embarrassed or affronted as she most certainly would have been had it been anyone else, she sat back, relaxed and settled in the chair.

Theodora was always asking Daisy to repeat herself, often feigning deafness to cover sporadic memory. When repeating, Daisy often got a sharp retort. Not so now. She didn't have to prove a thing, not with Jack, the great fountain of knowledge, incredibly by her side.

He was helping residents self-manage, as he was doing, all of what he'd developed to accommodate his near-absent sons. Still inclusive, he'd say, 'It's important that residents don't feel forgotten. A big factor that they are not shut away.' He himself had been. He overrode and created a life for himself to more than compensate for the loss of what no longer was.

For the relatives who did visit, Jack said, 'Ask what the resident wants to do. Most probably, they don't want to go out. If at home, visitors would probably visit in your lounge.'

Don't presume, thought Daisy. *Ask first. Good point.* The physio approach is to always get out and do something, but options and freedom of choice are as important at the end of the day.

'The main thing is that everyone feels comfortable and safe, that they are comfortable with their surroundings, where you can say what you want to say in a reasonable distance from others so there is that verbal space,' said Jack.

Mm, thought Daisy. *It doesn't take long before you forget what it is like on the outside. No privacy here.*

Once inside, everything was out in the open. You may be speaking quietly to someone sitting next to you, considered private, but in reality, every ear was straining. For the likes of Theodora, that was a bonus. She wanted everyone to know she was from a wealthy family and on the lookout for a man like Jack. And the likelihood was she had almost found one.

She now had her shopping list, no doubt for her daughter to acquire. *Soon it'll be lipstick*, Daisy thought.

Jack didn't have the luxury of shopping lists. He relied on his good deportment and intellectual acumen to get him through. So far, that was working a treat.

'It's important that it is positive, not negative,' said Daisy.

'Everything about here is positive,' said Jack. 'We have all the necessities. It's all positive, in fact. All our neighbours are in the same building. Family has just grown. That's it.

You just want in your room what you use, no point having furniture here you don't use. I don't like putting marks on the pristine walls. Fold-up photographs are enough.

'Being military trained, the less you have, the better, less to look after, less to clean. You just need a wardrobe, drawers, and a clock; a private room; a bed; three meals a day. All aspects of life are looked after.'

Well, that's it in a nutshell, thought Daisy. He was just as efficient in speech as in action.

Jack can get recalcitrant old ladies to sit in their chairs faster than any staffer can, even when they said, 'Are you getting a chair? Can you find another one?' meaning *Sit with me. I want you all to myself.*

It was 'Soon, love.' And he was on his way.

He was always giving up his seat up with a 'There we are, sweetheart. It's all nice and warm for you now.'

He never settled in one spot. It was a good way to avoid any unforeseen attachments and not have any extra demands put on you. He just kept moving, not the way Theodora liked it, but not having a choice in the matter, she had to accept it. He really covered the ground and did a lot of good. In between, it was to his room to lie down and think – ideal.

'I treat them as ladies, not as things,' said Jack. He refused to have favourites or take sides.

Everyone got frustrated with Mrs Cooper. She was constantly closing all the curtains, even on a sunny day, blocking the view and the last vestige of any outdoor reality they had. Residents got really feisty about it. Whenever they reopened them, she was at it again. Not Jack. Still, he gave her the 'How are you, sweetheart?' and a kiss on the back of the hand.

Theodora can't believe he can be so magnanimous. But on these matters, Jack remained unmoved. To win his favour, you had to accept his embracive approach, non-negotiable, as Beverly, now unwell, had to learn. *Better than a thousand tolerance lessons*, Daisy thought.

Everyone gravitated to the lounge as they enjoyed the company. As said by Delilah, 'I think I like to sit here in the lounge. You are on your own enough anyway.'

What a comeback, Daisy thought.

Now wearing trim black pants and sporting a brand-new haircut, Delilah was looking quite the part. The family must have come on board. It was an incredible difference to her previously forlorn state where she looked as if she was about to gladly depart this mortal world. Now smiling and with her sarcasm practically evaporated, she was a pleasant person to be around.

Someone was showing an interest. What a difference. She was even keen for Daisy to take an iPhone photo of her so she could see herself. Good on her. Residents never got to see themselves. All they had was the mirror above the handbasin, so they only got to see themselves shoulders up. Imagine trying to keep your body image intact with only your head and shoulders to go on.

Thankfully, the Filipino staff made a great effort in dressing residents well, coordinating colours etc. Otherwise, they'd have no show. Variety in clothing made a difference. A decent wardrobe helped. It made it easier for carers to mix and match. Residents had forty to fifty people pass them by on any given day, all staff and visitors taken into account. So being presentable made a difference. It got noted.

More and more, Daisy was seeing positive signs of socialisation happening – helping one another, having engaging, intellectual discussion, enjoying one another's company. It seemed everyone was happy, but Daisy thought she better confirm it. She liked to check in regularly to ensure she was on track.

At the next workshop group, with eight participating, she said, 'I want to find out how happy you are with things. There is a gradient of nought to ten to give feedback on. If you are happy, say ten. If unhappy, say nought. If middling, say five. So how do you feel about your rooms?'

Ignoring the scale, all said, 'Happy.'

'How do you feel about your whole accommodation, lounge, and dining area?'

All said, 'Happy.'

'And with one another?'

All said, 'Happy.'

Well, that confirmed that in a hurry, Daisy thought. *Going well.* Of course, that could change later in the day; but more and more, she observed that the well-socialised residents were maintaining a stable, happy mood.

Attempting to sum it up in her congenial manner, Patsy said, 'You look around here. It's well kept, clean. Everything's good. People are doing what they are meant to be doing. Everyone is pleasant to one another.'

And Jack said, 'I have a lot of sisters around. You have the freedom to do what you want here. There are new faces coming through the door. You feel part of the community. This is our community, all at the same address. We are relaxed and comfortable. Can relax just like at home. It's important to fit in.'

And the latest resident, Win, stated, 'I have a nice little room, a lovely little room. I'm very happy here. We are all friends.'

More and more, the new residents were having positive experiences, paving the way for others and setting the tone of the community. Daisy was hoping Jack would stay the way he was and not hook up with anyone else too quickly. Fortunately, he was open that Bev was his wife. But unfortunately, her health had gone down markedly, and she was now in line to go over to the hospital. It would be sad seeing her go. Such an independent spirit honed from the outback.

Having Jack at the unit was great company for the women. Most of their husbands died long ago, and some hadn't had any decent male company for decades. So a nice 'good morning' and a bit of a chat went a long way.

'It's a community here, and we are all Europeans. If you look at it, looking around, when you think about it, we are all the same age. We have all had the same history. All these factors are a conversation point – same upbringing, same surroundings, same parenting. It's a big symphony. Seventy-five per cent here are widowed grannies,' he says.

12

Glass Half Full

'Half the senior doctors on the front lines of our public health system are at breaking point,' Daisy read.

'Because they're very bright, they don't realise it,' said Theodora.

'Even your surroundings can give you mental stress. You need peace and quiet to reduce it. Stress doesn't show, not like measles. You have to look for the signs,' said Jack.

'All this background noise can increase stress,' said Theodora.

'It can often be a person sitting quietly in the corner, buried in their own thoughts. You have to recognise the symptoms, like them sitting there by themselves, looking out the window quietly. Some people don't know how to converse with other people,' he said.

'Not wanting to converse with anyone', she replied.

'We could have the classes on stress. We don't recognise it. You don't even recognise it in yourself. A lot of symptoms are illusive. You lose the art of communication. If you discuss it, it releases the mental energy. Otherwise, it can become a top hat of problems. At least we are discussing it now. When we discuss it, it becomes less of a problem,' said Jack.

'Depression and breakdown. Breakdown is another thing altogether,' she said.

'John Kirwan has been a great ambassador for depression,' said Daisy.

'That was good, wasn't it?' said Theodora. 'Very good.'

'Problem with depression is you can't recognise it,' said Jack.

'You can recognise depression if you read enough,' quipped Theodora.

'If mentally weak, you are vulnerable. People pick up on that and use it against you, bullying.'

'That gives depression.'

'Look at those brains,' said Theodora.

'My head will get bigger and bigger,' he joked.

'Some get embarrassed,' she continued.

'Another point is you can't find the right words to describe it,' he said.

Thelma said, 'Sometimes compared with others, you might appear weak. I'm always aware of you, Jack, because you are always talking.'

'The art of ageing', he said.

'Ageing mentally well. A lot of them lose their marbles once they start ageing unfortunately. I don't suppose that has happened to you. You're so perfect in every way.'

'Yeah, if I shake my head, I can hear the marbles rattling around.' He laughed.

'I don't mean to interrupt you,' said Josephine when Daisy asked if she'd mind not chattering to Dorothy in the group session. 'I find it very interesting.'

'I do too,' said Dorothy, sitting next to her.

Daisy thanked her for befriending Josephine and including her in the group. Previously, she'd just sat at a distance, not having the confidence to join in.

'I don't mind doing that,' said Dorothy. 'Neighbours were always asking me to quieten down little Johnny. I've always done babysitting for my sisters. I'm one of seven,' she said.

'Listening is learning,' said Jack.

What a great dialogue this has been, Daisy thought. *Best yet.*

It was mid-afternoon. David had just completed the jigsaw of *The Boat Builders* by Winslow Homer in record time. Daisy was happy for him. He deserved it. He'd had a rough week with Marina and had just said to Daisy, 'I'll lose my temper, and that won't be a good thing.'

Now he was king of the castle. The puzzle was laid out, perfectly placed, every piece. He was beaming. Proudly explaining his process, he said, 'Everything fits nicely. It's done. Didn't take too long. That has cleaned it up. Hello. It's all working. Do you know what? I really enjoy these things, like I did in business. I built it back, and it worked.'

Buoyed by his new-found sense of accomplishment, David confidently strode over to the exercise class that Daisy was now taking. He took to the floor with ease and started wiggling his hips to 'It's a Long Way to Tipperary'. He was having a great time centre stage.

Christina, by now, was doing her usual trick of lying supine on the coffee table, abdomen protruding; she liked to eat others' meat meals, even though she was down as vegetarian. With grace, David took both her hands, got her up, and started dancing. She started mouthing the words to the songs. 'Look, she is talking. She is talking,' David said excitedly, having never witnessed it as indeed no one else had. That she was mouthing the words to the song rather than talking didn't matter. It was the time for achievements to be acknowledged. And he was right there, front and centre, in the thick of it.

'I want to make an announcement. I want to thank you all for . . .' He trailed off at this point, so Daisy filled in with 'David has just completed a jigsaw puzzle about boats and wanted to thank you all for the support of his achievement. Is that right, David?'

'Yes, it is. It definitely is,' David said enthusiastically.

Amidst this, Theodora said, 'I'd like to see your boats.'

Oh dear, thought Daisy. *She better be nice.*

Aiming to raise David's profile for status-conscious Theodora, Daisy quickly said as she sped by, 'He sailed his own boat all across the Mediterranean.'

'Oh really', she said, suitably impressed.

Daisy wasn't sure if David could find his way over to the nurses' station, let alone locate the jigsaw puzzle. Did he have the orientation for that? He did. He found it. And there was Theodora right beside him, leaning over the waist-high mahogany nurses' station, stretching herself up, peering over the edge. There it was, shimmering in its glory.

'That's fantastic,' said Theodora, giving ample encouragement.

Good on her, Daisy thought, concerned that it could have gone the other way.

Something is in the air, she thought. She could feel it.

Just a few hours before, Daisy had gone down to Theodora's room to remind her that the press reading was on. Putting on her pearls, Theodora was in an especially jubilant mood as she made her way down the corridor. Uncharacteristically, she said, 'Can I help with anything?' Daisy couldn't believe what she was hearing. Then she quickly qualified with 'Tell me quickly before I become mean again.'

It seemed Theodora's scornful ways were modifying, at least in part. She'd obviously laid it on for David. Her intelligence and dramatic flair made her praise all the more salubrious. It was carrying weight, and she was sailing on the waves of her new-found charitable status.

Buoyed by this, she thought she'd press her luck further with the ubiquitous Jack. Now perched dangerously at the edge of her walker seat, her spinal scoliosis was nowhere in sight. Bedecked with her new stick of Mary Quant lipstick and long string of pearls, she said, 'I want to sit on Jack's knee.'

Jack, delighted, was thumping his thighs with resounding encouragement. Theodora was already lurching her way across the exercise class when she was quickly pulled back and restrained by a vigorous staff member. 'I have an announcement to make too,' said Theodora. 'She just told me that I'm too heavy to sit on Jack's knee and for me not to sit on my walker like this. But if I fall, I don't care. I'll take responsibility for it!'

The whole place was breaking out in pandemonium. Even Mrs Cooper was clapping and shouting out some loud Chinese incantations. Staff were aghast. What was happening? Party time, that was what. They had just broken all the boundaries, dancing with one another rather than with staff, perching precariously on walker seats, lurching over to sit on one another's knees, hooting, cheering, swirling hips.

Once the exercise class was over, David said, 'It's good to have fun, isn't it? No one's being harmed.' Daisy thought the same, but ever-cautious staff didn't always agree.

The outbreak restrained, staff took residents mechanically and methodically to dinner. Things were never going to be the same again. They'd broken out once. They'd try it again. Their voice was building, not one of anger and violence now but one of espousing rights and challenging authority. The weekend staff were more lenient so had let the behaviour go. But such rule breaking in the week may not be tolerated with the more autocratic full-time staff.

Daisy stayed late, doing her notes, often the case. It had been a busy day.

At dinner, Gabrielle went wild, not uncommon, chaotically throwing plates of food all around the dining room. Quick-acting staff saved residents from harm. There was, though, one casualty.

From her workstation, Daisy heard a familiar voice say, 'Ow. That hurts. Someone just hit me over the back of the head!' It was Theodora. Daisy went over.

'She shouldn't be here,' she complained.

'Gabrielle's being reassessed, Theodora. But it takes time to get transfer and placement organised.'

'Well, I'm making a complaint. Whom do I talk to?'

'The unit manager, coming in tomorrow.'

Daisy hoped she'd remember. She told the unit manager about it and suggested she talk to Theodora about it to give some reassurance. But the nurse said Theodora hadn't said anything to her so just left it at that.

If this had happened to someone outside, it would have been taken much more seriously. Here, the resident was more or less just expected to put up with it as the staff so often did. Staff were thinking that residents would forget about it anyway, so they didn't treat it as such a big thing. But post-traumatic stress is a very real thing, good memory or not. And how can someone feel safe again, having been hit over the head from behind in their very own lounge?

After the incident, Theodora was remarkably cool, saying, 'It's easy to just sit here and fall away.'

'It's all about feeling safe and being part of the community,' said Daisy.

'Absolutely', said Theodora.

Changing topic, Theodora said, 'I always knew she was intelligent,' referring to Juliette sitting next to her. Juliette was certainly becoming much more eloquent, so Theodora's comments were not unfounded.

Theodora had spent a lot of time schooling her on the names of her five children. Initially, she could only get one, her youngest son, Daniele, her most regular visitor. But after their ample question and answer sessions, Juliette could now rattle off all five with ease. It was Theodora's initiative entirely. As a former schoolteacher, her tutoring was still up to speed; but so far, the only one she had tried it with was Juliette.

'It's now refining it,' said Theodora.

'Isn't it. The work.'

'Exercise is important too,' said Juliette. 'We can be happy at this age and have a lot of fun.'

So yes, all pieces of the pie needed to be there.

The next day, Suzie visited. Daisy updated her on David's accomplishments – the puzzles, the speeches, the caring for the ill, and the help with Iven, the blind man. Iven's wife always appreciated David's help. She'd already said to Daisy, 'It doesn't feel right to me, only coming to see him twice a week as I was told to do so as to let him settle. It doesn't feel right. I know him. After all, I've been with him for sixty-six years.'

Daisy had to be careful not to be seen to be going too much against the staff advice so just said, 'You know best.'

Daisy went back to talk to Suzie. She said the main problem, since David stopped working, was the lack of productivity. 'Yes, I've worked since I was 15,' David piped in.

'I can figure it out. If it is not fitting in properly, I ask them, "What do you think of it?" Put it back on them. Next conversation, I say that "I notice you did this, said this and this." Then we can work it out,' said David.

'He's excelling here,' said Suzy. He had been high up in the service and won awards. It meant a lot to him. He always worked hard. Having purpose here helps.'

Soon after Suzy left, David wanted to phone her again, asking Daisy to liaise. The nurse wasn't keen to call so soon after she'd just visited. Daisy went over and updated him. 'I have broad shoulders. I can handle it. I'll wait for tomorrow,' he said cheerfully. 'Just so I can clarify so I won't make mistakes.' This wish to clarify could be from a subconscious flash back that he wasn't able to remember specifically.

The previous week, David had lost it with Marina. She'd been pestering him all day, and he was well over it. She just wouldn't give up. He'd said 'I don't want you around' and 'get out' as many times as he could, but she still kept mincing around, unperturbed. Wherever he sat, she'd shadow him, sitting in the chair directly opposite. Not as garish as before, she'd now taken on a more low-key, subtle approach, so it was not as apparent to staff that it was still such a significant problem.

David was walking around the corridor with his son, with Marina trailing behind. Provoked beyond belief, he lunged at her, launching into a flood of vulgar profanities. His son was shocked, having never witnessed such, and had to quickly restrain him, luckily for Marina and fortunately for David having sympathetic family members to support.

Suzie said he felt terrible afterwards. He knew that something had happened, but he couldn't remember what. So when he'd said to Daisy the previous afternoon, 'I can lose my temper, and that won't be a good thing,' he was still aware that he could lose it and aware of the repercussions of his actions. That he was still making such a concerted effort to constrain himself Daisy admired.

The previous three men at the unit of David's size and build hadn't been so lucky. Unable to restrain themselves, they'd been medicated up and shipped off as a result. That David was able to tolerate on most occasions was testament to his strength of character and his family's support. Not easy in 24/7 confinement. He was very lucky that his son was there to restrain him as big strong men can do a lot more damage, and it didn't go down well when written up in the charts.

Nevertheless, amidst all the violating, it had been a good day. That same morning, Helena's daughter had visited. She was ten years younger than most, which helped, but it was the devoted care of her husband, Stephen, that made all the difference. He took her out for daily walks and was always attentive when visiting. They had always loved the outdoors and hiked everywhere and often. Even though it was a very scaled-down version now, the principle remained the same. They never missed a day.

The daughter, who rarely visited – as she lived a one-hour flight away – said, 'I've just had a lovely morning with Mum.'

'In what way?' said Daisy.

'Mum is so animated, happy. She has been telling me stories of when we were younger. She is looking younger, more beautiful every year. It's her personality too. She is always been about half glass full rather than half glass empty.'

13

Time Out

Many of the ladies sat all day in the lounge. Having no cosy room to go back to, they frequently escalated stress-wise. If it was cold, dark, and damp in their personal quarters, then it is the lounge that they'd opt for. 'You need to be prepared psychologically and emotionally. Everyone comes to such a place, don't they?' said Jack.

'I'll just go to my room,' said David as he hustled past the nurses' station. Marina had been provoking him all day, and the other ladies he'd been trying to help had just kept escalating. Rather than ratcheting right up there with them, he knew that lying down in his room was going to serve him better than anything else. Good at assessing his needs, he's garnered others' respect.

In his room, he didn't want for much – a few photos of the family, a couple of awards, a new duvet with the ocean blue all over it, and the crown jewel, his wardrobe. Suzie liked him well dressed, all good labels and fit for a king. Being tall, he suited the lot.

Daisy admired David. Initially suicidal, he had worked hard at creating a life for himself and harnessing his pent-up emotions. She witnessed mild aggression only once when Marina was trailing and hassling; he brushed her off with a 'get off me, will ya?' So she hadn't seen David in the aggravated state when his son had to restrain him. Daisy thought David's efforts admirable when he could have easily created more chaos like his predecessors of similar size and strength. They'd throw themselves around and frequently attack staff and residents. David's outbursts were only when provoked and only with Marina and a rare occurrence. He wouldn't hit anyone as others had.

It was incredible how five-foot-nothing Filipinos can manage these massive men. No security here, not even a male staff member a lot of the time.

David's self-developed tolerance and patience served him well when attending to the sick and dying. Sitting for hours, he'd never so much as skip a minute of his self-proclaimed duties. He had a natural compassion and concern.

Spiritual calm and solace was sorely absent for many. Devout residents often said, 'I've always been to church, and now I never get to go.' They were churchgoers all their life, and now they didn't get a chance. Though services were held over in the village hospital, residents needed an escort to take them. Previously, Daisy and staff had been able to, but that had been stopped much like the outside walks. Unless relatives took up the reins, the person didn't get there. And as services were midweek, few relatives were available anyway.

Special event inclusion was next to nil and socialisation with the rest of the village practically non-existent. It was a limited view in Daisy's opinion, considering many of them ended up staying there. 'Out of sight, out of mind' was the prevailing attitude.

Once firm friends with your neighbour in the village, now in the unit, it was rare that they visited. Husbands and wives were different, old school, loyal to the end. Witnessing the stigma that their partner was subjected to once admitted, many chose to opt for socialising at the unit. They were treated better there anyway. They can come and go as they pleased, welcomed and appreciated. Morning and afternoon tea were provided. They arrived just in time for that, like home away from home. Rather than battling away to be included in a community that had rejected them, it was better to create one of their own. Residents soon forgot what was over there anyway, even those with their partners still living there.

When invited over, they rarely wanted to go, even for the Anzac service. They had all the Anzac pageantry anyway – photos around the walls, poems read to them, a brilliant

Anzac service on the TV screen. And here, they got a front row seat with morning and afternoon tea provided in comfort, whereas over there you were always delegated to the back row, where you can hardly see a thing, and battling for a cup of tea served at ominous large tables was hardly worth the effort it took to acquire it.

'The residents enjoy being where they are if they are settled and comfortable,' said Jack. 'Everything about here is positive. We have all the necessities. You feel part of the community. This is our community, all at the same address. We are relaxed and comfortable. Can relax just like at home.'

Sometimes Daisy forget how hard it must be for the men. For all twenty-five women, there were only a handful of men and presently only two who can communicate with others effectively, David and Jack. David found it particularly difficult. Being a former detective, he was used to de-escalating situations and working out practical solutions. He had always enjoyed a high success rate in his work and attempted to do the same here. Some ventures were more successful than others. It was not always easy for him, especially with the women who kept ranting and raving, no matter what his efforts to pacify them.

Jack, by contrast, had mastered the art of meet-and-greet. He was an expert at hotfooting it onto the next seat so he didn't get caught up in the maelstrom, whereas David sat there indefinitely, as long as it took, ready for the long haul, intent on getting a solution. Often, it was a long time in coming. You could be at the end of your tether by the time it arrived.

David's tolerance got tested to the max, more difficult as his elocution wasn't as well honed as Jack's. That along with his thick Irish accent often made him difficult to understand. People often attempted to brush him off, not thinking he had anything worthwhile to contribute.

Persevering with 'I want to help', to his credit, he wouldn't let up. Those lying in the recliner chair certainly needed it, the quiet, unwell ones not likely to be with us much longer.

But the screeching women – he was beginning to realise that he wasn't the one to help them. He was with a day resident called Ursula. Feigning deafness but hearing when she wanted to, she complained and moaned from the minute she was dropped off by her daughter at nine in the morning till when picked up again at five in the afternoon. Her voice had a serial siren whine to it, on all day. He brought her by the hand to Daisy, saying, 'She needs help. She needs help now!'

Daisy tried to explain, 'She is well cared for, David, and her daughter is picking her up at five o'clock. There really isn't a problem.'

Finally, David came to his own conclusion. 'I don't want to sit by her anymore.' He chose instead to sit in the nurses' hub, doing his puzzles. It was more peaceful and a good respite, garnering him a formidable concentration. Daisy actually got to like sitting next to him, especially when doing long reports, the direct opposite of her initial stance. Thinking he'd take up too much time and she wouldn't get through her work, she was proved wrong. He has proved to be an amiable asset.

David's partner, Suzy, visited regularly, alternate days at least. And she had a long drive to get there. She was great. She took David out, lots of walks. She drove out in the car, had cups of tea at the unit, and joined in activities. Nothing was too much trouble. It was not always easy as she was very fit and sporty, and here was a very different pace. She had to slow herself right down. Sometimes biting her tongue, whatever was good for David, she'd go with that.

Her big asset was her accessibility. She never blocked phone calls, always available. David can call her whenever he wished, and staff regularly put calls through. She had grown to like the unit and the residents in it.

It was incredibly stressful when David first arrived though. All he wanted to do was go home and be with her. He had nothing else on his mind. 'I just want to be with my Suzy,' he'd call out morning, noon, and night.

Her pitch was, 'David, you are here to get your sleeping patterns sorted.' It was a good approach as he knew his sleeping was all over the place. She'd tried taking him home, but he was up all night, and none of them had any sleep. So it ended up being an exhausting experience for everyone. Best to take things day by day.

Local and often worked out best to the unit. They mixed in, socialised, and were out and about when they were both in the mood for it. Once Suzy had gone, David was back to the nurses' station. Focusing on the job at hand, he can sit there for hours, no pain, no anguish, no mourning for Suzie as before, just the puzzle and him. He was working it out. He got plenty of passing comments. 'Haven't you finished that yet?' roared Nan.

Nell, ever encouraging, said, 'You're doing really well,' and even, 'You are more alert,' meant as an encouragement from the charge nurse.

David didn't mind, unfazed. If relatives came through the front door, he flamboyantly waved them over to the charge nurse. Otherwise, he had his space, and he was sticking to it.

He was one of the lucky ones. Not everyone got to sit in the nurses' hub. Coveted seats were prizes. Only eight sunny seats were available at the window alcoves, ten front row seats for the workshops, plenty, though, for the second row, which expanded back into the dining room. That was why Daisy had to throw out her voice to be heard and hoped she hadn't wrecked her larynx in the process.

No matter where they were sitting, there was one activity that everyone got a chance in – singalong. They can join in from anywhere. If they didn't sing, they mouthed the words at least. 'Daisy Daisy, of course, was the favourite. They loved that – everyone except Theodora. 'Oh no, not "Daisy Daisy".

I can't stand it!' She preferred Bach, which she played ably on her piano each morning.

Residents knew Aunt Daisy from her famous radio programme in the forties and fifties. The namesake song was sung before each of her morning shows, where she'd espouse entertainingly, everything a housewife needed for a modern home. The song graced kitchens for decades, part of the residents' generational DNA. So when singing, in tune mostly, it was a great solace, memorable, enjoyable, fun, and achievable.

Sometimes you aren't really sure what will work until you try it. But 'Daisy Daisy was always a hit. The veranda not so, at least initially.

Conscientious attempts were made to make it attractive and accessible so people would go out there to relax and enjoy the sun. It didn't work. Hardly anyone went out there, only the wanderers. Even with the newly planted begonias and daffodils, colourful outdoor cushions, the newly painted wheelbarrow, and the evermore ornate garden ornaments, nothing happened, not until two very sturdy things were bought into the mix.

These were a hugely strong and stable umbrella which gave easily enough shade for four, eight at a squash, and a comfortable set of high-quality garden furniture, two chairs and a table. The chairs were admirably light and fortuitously easy to move around. All of a sudden, everyone was out there. Now you could hardly get a seat on a sunny day. It just took those two things and a few fragrant bushes of nice-smelling lavender to completely change the space. Now sacred, it was time out for everyone – except Nell, David's friend.

She was not so keen, never really adjusted. She spent most of the time in her room. Her daughter spent a lot of time on it, and the resultant feng shui was palpable. With her good view, a nice set-up, and David being right next door, it suited her just fine, as best as it can be anyway. Although the patients were good, they were not her cup of tea, except of course David, whom she spent a lot of time with.

Her daughter was very attentive and took her out for coffees and brunches practically daily, so she didn't really need to mix in with the others too much. She had her room, her books, and her view. David and her daughter were enough socialising for her.

Daisy always liked to see the rooms well set up. They were big enough to be able to make them nice and cosy, so it seemed a waste not to, especially for those who spent a lot of time in them. Making them homely was one of the best things a family can do in her opinion.

Bernie also had a great set-up but with none of Nell's advantages, neither a good outlook nor a sunny spot. It was cold and dark on that south-facing side, and most relatives did little to ameliorate it, often not spending enough time in there to know what it was like. Not so with Bernie. Her vivacious florist daughter had it all sorted out, with the heater on all the time so dry, warm, and no damp; TV going but low volume so just enough for background company; a comfy two-seater for Bernie and guests to sit on; always fresh flowers in the room; a big bureau with lots of favourite ornaments; and a light on a stand in the corner, out of the way, shedding a natural neon ambience.

Her bed was colourful and cosy – a duck down duvet, a blue mohair rug, two feather pillows. Perfect. It was always comfortable to lie on any time of the day or night. Bernie was as happy in her bedroom as she was out in the lounge. She had the best room on the south side.

Many of the ladies sat in the lounge all day long, having no cosy room to go back to where they can lie down in comfort and relax. These were those ladies who ended up escalating with stress, the ranting and raving ones whom David was trying to deal with. They were getting no quality time out. If it was cold, dark, and damp in their personal quarters, then it was the lounge that they'd opt for.

'You need to be prepared psychologically and emotionally, to prepare your thinking pattern. Need to get acclimatised. Familiarisation, everyone comes to such a place, don't they? When you can't mow the lawns or do the garden anymore, you know you are going to have to go somewhere else soon. It is better to be prepared. As you get older to think, "Where will I live?" to think what is next, develop a positive mindset. Boy Scout motto, "Be prepared",' said Jack. 'It's not only our voice. It's for the future residents, to prepare them as they get on in years. The work is for the future residents, preparing for the future.'

*   *   *

Daisy was able to speak to Janet just a couple of days before she died. She'd been relegated to the recliner. On being told about the residents' comments being written up in a manuscript, her eyes lit up. 'We have to put it in writing as we have to create an impression in the long term so people don't have to start doing it all over again.'

Janet had been the initiator of this Residents' Progress Mission Statement: *Everyone is becoming much more humane. There are people who are not. But they will catch up in time. Everything is getting back to* reality.

14

Report

The breakthrough in the dementia work is best explained in the following report on which all work in this book is based and built. It is a formal account I sent to Bill Gates's Intellectual Ventures Lab in Seattle but important reading to understand the depth and detail behind the work.

Activating Intelligence within Dementia

This involves the engagement of the intellect rather than trying to pursue the path of the restricted memory component of the mind. This breakthrough is psychological, not pharmaceutical.

At the dementia facility where I work, most have advanced Alzheimer's disease. Six years ago, these residents were very low functioning, shut down and shut off from both themselves and one another. They had virtually no communication of any sort.

Now they are readily engaging both individually and in the group, right through from morning to night. They are creating a confident literary culture all of their own. Library books, workshops, quizzes – they just can't get enough. How on earth did this massive turnaround happen?

To explain, end of 2015, I'd been working at the unit for almost a year. I'd tried practically everything, but nothing had really engaged the residents up to that point. So Friday, 4 December, the end of that same year, I decided to do something completely different. I wheeled the whiteboard in and, on the off-chance, wrote up, 'There is nothing either good or bad, but THINKING makes it so' (*Hamlet*).

Then something amazing happened. From being totally shut down, with literally no conversation, to that point, the residents started to engage, make constructive comments, and converse. It was the THINKING part they liked. For a solid hour, they THOUGHT about and discussed that one line. What is good, what is bad, and how does thinking make it so?

Then I started to think, 'How is it that minds with dementia, which are meant to have no advanced thinking capacity at all, are able to reason and communicate in this way?' I couldn't speak to any of my friends like this, not on Shakespeare anyway, and certainly not for this length of time.

Then it dawned on me . . . slowly at first. The residents who have been diagnosed with dementia have a WORKING INTELLECT. And it can be engaged and activated. They just need to be given the chance and then educated and encouraged!

The existence of the intellect is well known, but how it can be activated with people with dementia is the revelation. It's all about the intellect part of the consciousness, separate to the mind, and training the intellect to think to take you through how to activate the intellect. It can initially be perceived as heavy going for relatives, but for residents who only have their intellect to work through, it's a salvation.

Residents love topics that are intellectually stimulating and anything to do with history, geography, psychology, and philosophy. In the lessons, each resident's name and their comment on the topic is written in big letters on the whiteboard. This has proved to be of great benefit.

The residents can still read. This is often not realised. They can read, and they love to read. They just need encouragement. The whiteboard compensates for their memory impairment by them being able to read, repeatedly if they wish to, in a relaxed way what they or one another have just said.

As in any form of thinking education, the individual has to 'want to do it'. You can't 'do it for them'. The thoughts can't be 'pushed in'. A culture of learning has to take place which is enjoyable, fun, disciplined, and eventful for everyone to want to join in. As the residents' interest increases and concentration grows, the impact is visible in their eyes – their relatives comment frequently on their 'blazing eyes and bright-eyed interest'.

Their motivation is high. It either is achieved through the channels of the intellect to control their 'fuzzy brain, fuzzy mind' or succumbs to the much publicised effect and consequences of extreme memory loss and lack of orientation.

Residents need to understand and know what's going on around them to have a starting point to move forward from.

One resident, whom I tutored privately for two years, has contributed enormously to the work. From this, she has been able to tell me, even amidst her 'fuzzy brain' episode, how the 'fuzzy mind' immobilises. From her explanation, I was able to start understanding how a person with dementia thinks.

An example of high interest and stimulation for another resident is with an ex-nurse, one of three nurses in the group. At this particular lesson, she said to me, 'Why do you keep tapping here? Between your eyes?"

I said, 'This is where you need to focus to engage and activate your intellect. It's the intellect that does the thinking, and this is where it is located. Through this thinking, you will be able to function and manage so much better.'

She said, 'I'll take that. It's been a long time since I've been shown something. Thank you'.

Then the other residents, listening to this, said, 'Yes, we like to learn.'

The extent of the residents' ability to learn and engage through the intellect depends to a certain extent on the individual – how they've lived, how they think, their fitness, their health, their resilience, their outlook, and their support network – but regardless, all residents receive benefit through this intellect work. There is no person with dementia who cannot receive benefit through this.

With the teaching itself, a lot depends on the energy and 'spark' the teacher/trainer creates. For this intellect work to be recognised and understood by the resident, one needs to develop a good rapport, be energised and enthusiastic, and have a friendly, engaging manner for the intellect to be activated to its fullest extent. Regardless, the path to the intellect is the vehicle uncovered to breach unchartered territory within dementia and to remove the problems of restlessness, helplessness, and feelings of being lost and isolated so often felt by those affected with such advanced memory loss conditions and other related issues.

This work and information enables not only the lives of the residents to be transformed but also, by association, the lives of their close family and friends. Residents' previously unheard voice of discontent and restlessness can be replaced with hope, self-worth, and feeling that there is genuine recourse for them, their opinions still matter, they are being heard, and their voice is getting louder. In the teaching sessions, there is competition for front row seats as both the second and third rows want to come closer, and relatives as well often like to attend.

One of the big gains of intellect engagement is an improvement in tolerance. This has had a profound effect in the unit. As a result of the increased tolerance levels, incident reports in aggression have reduced markedly and with that the need to medicate or, as is sometimes the case, over-medicate.

Here is an example of how this has worked. Front row residents used to get very impatient with the wanderers as the wanderers would come into the group, take their walkers, walk all over their feet, and generally get in the way. The front row would often overreact to them. At times, it could get quite heated. So there were lots of tolerance lessons to calm the waters, so to speak.

The additional education on this one point has had a big spin-off effect. The front row started to develop more understanding, compassion, and insight for the others in the unit, including the wanderers. Their changed attitude has introduced a new culture of friendship and kindness. As noted by all, residents feel more at home. Relatives find the unit more relaxed, and staff are grateful that all the residents get to join in and feel included.

The work and training approach has been both well documented and self-funded by myself to date and is now becoming recognised and acknowledged to an increasing degree by those both within the unit and outside. My medical family have also supported me, especially my father, an enlightened primary care physician in his time who focused on self-management skills and a blend of physical and mental fitness within his practice, similar to what I instituted in my former physiotherapy practice of twenty years.

Thank you for your consideration in reading this report.

Regards,
Pieta Valentine diversional therapist
(recreational therapist)
Former physiotherapist

Epilogue 1

Entry in to the Unit

The following points and techniques are for relatives to best help their loved one going into a dementia unit. It is derived from the author's observational skills and experience from thirty-five years as a physiotherapist both in New Zealand and in England, Canada, and Australia, working with geriatrics for ten of those years and her private practice work of twenty-five years treating workplace injuries for stress and neck and shoulder pain. This and a range of supportive attitudes and actions from relatives and residents at the unit has contributed to the following points and perspectives.

The scenarios quoted are the case for the various dementia units the author has worked in but may vary in other dementia facilities. The intention of these pointers is to outline important points to you that you aren't as likely to find on Google or any other reading material more readily available on the subject.

With the points outlined below, it is assumed that the relative will include the resident in the decision-making processes that affect them if they are able, especially in terms of their room set-up and dietary choices.

Forms

The power of attorney (POA) will be asked to fill out a vast range of forms. All are important. In particular, the forms for activities must be filled out in detail: the names of the children, the husband or wife, the birthdays, the anniversaries, the common visitors and good friends, and their interests. Do they like walking or not? What sort of music do they like? Do they read the newspaper? Are they an extrovert or an introvert? What company do they like? Male, female, or both? Do they like to go to church; if so, which church?

The answers to these questions are taken seriously by the activities coordinator and staff to best develop a portfolio that best fits the resident. The special details are important.

POA and Phone Calls

The POA plays a big role in the resident's care and quality of life. They will be the main person of contact. It is good to put forward another phone number of someone easily available or close to the resident, especially if you are not readily available, not just for emergencies but also for the resident to phone (put through by the nurse) when they are stressed or wanting to speak to someone. The best scenario when the nurse rings is for it to be answered straight away as they are really busy. They can then hand the phone straight to the expectant resident.

Siblings

The POA is a big role for anyone whose parent is in a dementia unit. There is a lot involved. It is important that it's not just left to one person.

Help from siblings is essential with such things as regular visits to the unit and help with appointments such as the dentist or a hairdresser off-site or buying a pair of shoes or a new hearing aid. It all helps share the load.

Getting to Know the Staff

There are a lot of people to get to know. So it is best to have a bit of an idea about what to expect before you go in as outlined below.

The initial contact person may well be the village manager. She will show you around and give you the overall rundown on things. You will only be dealing with her again on important matters. It is the dementia unit itself that you need to get familiar with day to day.

Top of the pyramid in the unit is the unit manager. She deals with all matters of importance. She runs the unit overall.

The charge nurse will act as the unit manager if they are off duty. Go to them regarding medications, appointments, medication when taking them out, dietary requirements, questions on increase or decrease of weight, questions on sleeping, eating, and socialisation, etc.

Each resident is appointed a full-time carer in most cases. It is really helpful for the resident if you get to know this person. Though most communication will go through the unit manager and charge nurse, it is the day-to-day showering, toileting, and cares that the carer is responsible for. Whilst all that information is recorded for the clinical manager and charge nurse to have at their fingertips, it is all about the personal touch. The carer deals with the resident daily. The carer won't approach you, but it is within your rights to approach them.

It is all about becoming part of the community at the unit and understanding what is going on. Most carers have nine residents to look after, so they are very busy but generally happy to talk. Try to catch them at a time when you can see that they are a bit freer.

Learning Curve of First Visit and Security

It is a big learning curve for the relative as well as the resident when first coming into the unit. Once the forms are filled in, the best thing you can do is to sit with the now new resident to orientate yourself and them. Look around and learn. Take it all in. Observe who the residents are, who the staff are, and as much as possible who the regular visitors are.

It is obvious who the staff are as they are in uniform, but it is not always obvious who the residents are. Residents can look in a better state than some relatives visiting, and as a result of this and by mistake, they are sometimes let out. This creates huge problems. Make sure this doesn't happen to you.

The charge nurse and staff are always on the lookout for escapees, but this can happen. Sit, watch, and observe those who are most likely to do this. They are often at the door, either banging incessantly on it or fiddling at the code. Try to get out the door when they are not there. Otherwise, ask a staff member to divert them while you exit. They will assist.

Being courteous and empathetic to all concerned is the best approach. Don't get upset if you are mistaken by another relative as a resident when you are leaving. It is all part of the course and best to take it in good humour.

Security Code

There will be a code you will have to learn to enter the unit and the same code for the lift, often four numbers followed by the hashtag. Bring a piece of paper to write it down on, enter it in to your phone, or one of the staff will write it down for you, and then memorise it.

Initial Visits

Often, relatives are advised to not visit for the first week and then to only come a couple of times a week so as to let the resident settle in. This can be very distressing for both parties. Those whose partners come daily or alternate days are more settled as a result.

Taking them out for a walk or a trip out in the car, if mobile enough, is good, especially if the resident themselves wants to get out. The only exception is if the resident is aggressive and if it is difficult getting them back into the unit after taking them out. Then trips out will need to be stopped until aggressiveness settles. This happens only in the minority of cases. The well-supported resident with a supportive family and friends will settle in and be a lot less stressed than those who don't.

Medication

Medication is a sensitive topic. Over-medication is to be avoided. If you find your mother or father, fit and active on entry to the unit, is now shuffling their way slowly along the corridor, then it could be the medication doing it. Permanent medication increases only happen with POA consent, so it pays to get upskilled.

It is important to develop good working relations with the unit manager, charge nurse, and doctor. As POA, you have the right to request a copy of your relative's notes, which staff will print out for you. Family meetings with the doctor are generally every three months (unless there has been a recent medical event), so be prepared and ask relevant questions so there can be robust discussion, and you can get thorough answers.

Epilogue 2

Room set up and Attire

The Room

Setting up the bedroom is a very important part of the resident's entry point into the unit. A room set up as close as possible to the one at home helps enormously in the settling-in experience and overall quality of life throughout the stay at the unit, which could be as long as five years, so it is important to make it cosy and not see it as temporary. Keep the set-up comfortable but not cluttered. Include items that you know are important to your relative that they will appreciate and engage with. There is a wide range here with common examples given below. Do not look at it as a temporary thing, but set it up as close to home as possible.

Getting a Room

Often, there isn't a choice, but a room with a view is the best option, especially if the person is an outdoors person; seeing a mountain scene or hills in the distance can be very reassuring and grounding. Similarly, for a gardener, looking out onto a bed of flowers brings much pleasure. Some are also just as happy seeing the coming and going of the cars. All this is ideal especially if the unit is up on a second storey where there is no possibility of getting outside independently.

Make sure that the main chair in the room is facing out towards the best view available and that furniture is not blocking the view. Readjust the chair's position if you find it has been changed next time you visit. The resident probably won't take the initiative to move it themselves, but once in position, they will sit in it and enjoy the view.

Lighting and Heat

A nice lamp adds ambience to a room, and it is amazing how much difference it makes to the overall atmosphere. Make sure it is not in a position where it is a tripping hazard. Especially if there is nice art or family photos on the walls, it really lifts the feel of the room from institutionalised to homely. Make sure your relative has a good-quality, safe, functional heater, especially in colder climates, in case the central system is not generating enough heat or if they are frail and need more heat.

The Chair

Bringing in the favourite armchair is absolutely vital. It is often the last vestige of home and an important one. It is where they will have spent most of their time watching the telly, looking out the window, knitting, or reading a book for many of them. It is tried and tested for comfort. It is worn to fit their shape. The colour, texture, and feel they like. It has all the good memories attached to it, so they can best relax in it.

It doesn't matter if the chair dominates the room. It is your relative sitting in it, so it is important that they are as comfortable as they can possibly be, especially if they have painful conditions such as rheumatoid or osteoarthritis. They need all the assistance they can get.

Visitors can sit on anything – a footstool, the bed, or another smaller chair – unless they are older, a sibling or spouse, and need a suitable chair as well. Space will need to be negotiated for that without the room getting too cluttered.

Just ensure that the height of the main chair is such that the person can get out of it independently. If not, check out if a suitably shaped foam cushion can raise the height to get to the right level. If that doesn't work, another chair from home may well do the trick. If not, buy a new one. It is the best investment, along with a good pair of shoes and glasses as explained later.

Last resort is to use the armchair already in the room. Not a good option though. They tend to be high and uncomfortable, more suitable for a boardroom and six-foot men than little old ladies of just five feet.

Bring in what you know is most comfortable for your relative, what they like, and what works. These are all important decisions as the rooms are small, and you don't want it to become too crammed as that can create a fall risk. But at the same time, you want it homely.

It is important for the person to be able to stand up from their chair because legs get a lot weaker as you get older, especially the large quadricep muscles at the front of the thigh. Residents have to have strong enough legs to independently get up and down from the chair, in and out of bed, and up from the toilet seat to be able to stay in such a facility. The person has to be independent in these particular activities of daily living. If not, then the person will be transferred to a higher level of care, either to a hospital where there is generally one carer to four or five residents or to a higher-level dementia facility.

Chair Accessories

Easier to transport and requiring less space in the room, the accustomed accessories around the chair (i.e. cushions, rugs, favourite books, pen and paper, knitting bag, and anything else that your relative commonly has at hand) are all important, valued items. These items will more likely keep the person oriented, having their own things around them, as well as aiding in comfort and interest.

Of course, there has to be enough space left for staff to move around and for it not to be too cluttered, especially if fall risks, but good strategic thinking can get around that. Take ideas from other well-set-up rooms on the floor and bring in furniture that fits and works best, ideally that the resident is familiar with.

Bed

It is important to have a favourite, familiar quilt or bed cover. It adds colour and texture to a room that can often otherwise look cold and bare. It is not about new and pristine but cosy and familiar.

Mohair rugs are great as they are light, colourful, and cosy.

Light duvets fit for a single bed work especially well, feather filled even better and of a nice warm colour. The reason is that the person can just lie down in the day and draw that over them easily, even if fully dressed. The unit's covers are often heavy and awkward down to the ground polystyrene bedspreads. They were too difficult to negotiate getting into for a nap and uncomfortable too. The mohair rug can also do as a throw-over to sleep under, but they need to be big enough to fit the full top of a single bed.

Make sure someone else washes them though. If they go through the company's laundry dryer, they will come back a matted mess (same for wooden cardigans).

Walls

Walls are the largest and most private space of the resident, so it is best to take advantage of them. They are private in the sense that it is rare that another resident will reach up to take something off them, especially if the items are higher up, whereas drawers are often pilfered by other confused residents thinking that it is their room.

Walls are fantastic for paintings of the farm, photo boards of the children, whiteboards for appointments and messages, kids' drawings, favourite art, etc. The maintenance department will hang them all up. Best to put a sticky and a number on the item and the same coloured sticky and number on the wall so the staff knows where to put them up. Rooms are generally repainted once the resident has left, especially if the resident has been there a long time, so any marks will be painted or plastered over.

Attaching a long mirror to the wall is a great help to assist with orientation and body image.

Photograph Memory Boards

Photographs in a collage form on a board, with names of people noted even better, attached to the wall act as a great conversation point. Some relatives write the names of the people on the glass of the bigger family photograph, again on the wall. Blown-up family and holiday photos with names added and Blu-Tacked up adds orientation, colour, and warmth to a room. All conversation points.

With the constant stream of carers (doing showering, toileting, and cares), cleaners (doing vacuuming, dusting, and rubbish), laundry staff (putting away the laundry), nurses (giving out medication), and carers again delivering morning and afternoon tea (if the person is lying down in their room), there are a lot of people coming and going, much more than you would ever have in your own home. 'All the girls coming in', as the residents put it, are a very important part of the resident's life, especially those who don't have visitors. They become like family. They are kind (otherwise, they wouldn't be working in the industry) and care for these people.

If there are photos on the wall, they will use them as a talking point to ask such things as 'Are they your grandchildren?' or 'Is that where you went for your family holiday?' This exchange is great for past memory prompting, conversation exchange, and friendship building.

Books, Magazines, and Bookcases

Even though the person may not be reading very much, it is always nice to have their favourite books around them to look at the familiar covers and flick through, especially photographs of the farm, tractors, cats, or dogs if that is what the person is interested in.

Bookcases are great as they go upwards, where there is the most available space, unlike the often cramped floor space below. They are an underrated piece of furniture for functionality. They are very much multipurpose in a place which is so short of room. Just make sure, if high, they are secured to the wall.

Everything from a bookcase is easy to reach and easy to see not only for the person in the room but also for wanderers. So make sure the items are not of high value but of visual and recreational value nevertheless. Anything can be put on them – books, magazines, jigsaw puzzles, photo albums, ornaments, religious artefacts, and vases of flowers. Magazines are a big deal for women. Just expect that they will be shared around. Books with a name on it will be kept in their room, but magazines tend to be seen as public property. The best way around that is to bring in a pile, plenty of spares. They don't have to be new. Gathering up old copies from friends and family and bringing them into the lounge is a great service to the community.

Doors Unlocked

Catholic women like to have a statue of Mother Mary in their room. Being heavy plaster of Paris, they are rarely carried off; and even if they were, they are easily found. Not so with small trinkets, ornaments, and jewellery.

Doors are not locked in a dementia unit, and the wanderers do go in and out of other people's rooms, picking up whatever catches their eye and planting it anywhere, often not found till a few months later; it is not malicious or intentional, but other residents often think that it is, and it can cause a lot of stress in the unit. It takes the staff a lot of time and energy trying to find these small things if lost. It is like looking for a needle in a haystack. Literally, it could be anywhere.

So for jewellery, costume jewellery is probably best, unless worn on the person as a wedding ring. Some relatives chose to bring in good-quality ornaments with the risk they'll go missing. If lost, it might just take time for them to be found again. They won't be going anywhere.

Walkers

Walkers can be both a blessing and a curse. They can be considered as a furniture item in the room as that is where they mostly live. They also act as a spare seat for many. They are a blessing in that they help with the resident's walking and as a handy side table for morning and afternoon teas. The curse is that they are a constant tripping hazard. So placement of them is paramount to prevent falls.

Staff often put them to the side so as to be out of the way, but it can then become a problem for when the person needs it. Walkers are always getting lost. Finding them can be a mission amidst the maze of other similar-looking vehicles. The best a relative can do is vamp it up so it is recognisable, much like people do for suitcases at an airport – ribbons, feathers, bells, photos, big name tags, a favourite ornament attached, anything to make it stand out both for the resident themselves and anyone else trying to find it. Initially, barcoded names are put on them, but they are in small print and often quickly peeled off.

Make the walker bright and easily seen if that is the personality of the resident, otherwise subdued and tasteful if that is more their style. But make sure to make it look different. So it can stand out. Be creative.

Walker baskets are very handy, especially for those who read. All their magazines, books, tissues, pens, paper (sticky note pads are good), chocolate, sweets, and other handy items can be put in there. Staff sometimes take them away as they get filled up with unnecessary items, like half the ornaments of their room. But if cleaned out and tidied by a relative, much like the drawers need to be, then the staff will not mind them.

A present, supportive relative always aids in keeping up the limited range of options available to the resident. No matter how small they may seem to us, for the resident who lives their life there, every bit of liberty helps.

Whiteboard

Some relatives leave diaries in bedrooms, and whilst a good intention, they can easily get lost. Better still, put up a secure whiteboard up on the wall near the bed below the light so the person can clearly see.

It is for appointments, keeping everyone in the loop. Future appointments written up aid as a fresh, new talking point for staff to engage in with the person, aiding in building up the all-important anticipatory feelings.

The other advantage is that residents are often able to read if eyesight is OK, especially if the writing on the whiteboard is in big clear print. So even though they can't remember, they can still keep updated. If written as *It is your birthday, 6 April. Ann is picking you up at 10 a.m.* the resident can read it and have the much-valued anticipatory feelings of looking forward to it. Otherwise, because of short-term memory loss, even if reminded, they forget and when picked up for the event are often shocked. With all the anticipatory reminding, they may not remember astutely about the event/appointment, but there will be a recognition it is about to happen, so they will better assimilate when it does.

Name and Photo Board on Door

With dementia, one of the first things to often go is orientation. Most have problems with it. Some have a good past memory but no direction orientation. It is a total mission every time they have to go to find their bedroom or bathroom, so any aid to find it is an advantage.

Many are short, and with being bent over a walking frame, their line of sight is often well below five feet. It is important for them to have their name and room number on their door at their line of sight so they can more easily read it when looking for their room. Often, their name and room number is up high, out of sight range, often above the jutting-out photo board, so they have no show of seeing it. It is suitable for a six-foot man but not for a five-foot-something stooped elderly woman. All that is needed is a laminated sign with their name and room number written in large letters and then Blue-Tacked to the door at eye level. This will save an enormous amount of distress for the resident trying to find her room.

Relatives are usually good at putting a recognisable photo in the wooden glass inset on the door, and that all helps with recognition, but the name and room number at the right height is the most important detail. The room number is generally quoted to the resident at the nurses' station when they are asking where their room is. So for that reason, it is important to have the room number on the sign and not just their name.

Residents have lots of stresses in their day-to-day lives. It is the relatives who look, listen, and learn on how to best help mitigate them.

Being Part of a Community

It is a community that your relative is entering. It doesn't have to be all doom and gloom, and it is best if not approached that way. Dementia units can be a lot of fun, and for the relatives who visit regularly, they begin to make friends with other relatives and become a part of the community as well.

Regularly visiting relatives are a great help at the unit. They get to know the ropes and can work out if something is serious or not. They can alert staff if someone has fallen or if they can see a fight breaking out. These interactions go a long way towards your relative's comfort and security. If you look out for another relative's family member, they, in turn, will do the same for you.

Shoes

Shoes, glasses, and hearing aids are expensive items, and they take time and effort to organise, but they make a huge difference to a resident's quality of life. A good pair of shoes can be the difference between being able to walk and not and between being able to stay in the unit and not. If the resident is unable to walk the required distances, it is off to the hospital or higher level of dementia care.

Shoes need to be properly fitted, taking into account arthritis, unstable joints, weaker musculature, bunions, and twisted toes that residents so often have. To get the best fit, take the person to a specialist shoe shop for elderly people, where they can fit the shoes properly. If a good pair of shoes can't be obtained, it is often slippers that become the default option. Trying to walk up and down long corridors in those, without the appropriate support around their feet, can often prove too much.

Good shoes give the person the best chance of counteracting gait problems. It is nice if they look good as well but not imperative.

Glasses

Most residents can read. They like to read, but they can't read unless they have recent subscription glasses provided for them. Glasses and hearing aids are kept in the nurses' station as they are expensive items and easily lost.

They need to be regularly cleaned. It is something a relative can do if the nurse is too busy. In case the carer has forgotten to bring them out, just go to the nurses' station, and they will bring them out for you.

Hearing Aids

Hearing aids can be easily lost. Consider carefully if purchasing a second pair. There is a lot of background noise at the unit which some hearing aids function poorly in. Also, many don't like wearing them. Speaking clearly and enunciating well while facing the person is all important.

Hairstyles and Outfits

Residents are as class conscious as anywhere, and an uncared-for, unkempt-looking person is dismissed as easily as anyone. Most facilities have a hairdressing salon on-site, and the weekly hair set is enjoyed by most, depending on their previous hairdressing history. Some just prefer a cut, and that's it. It is important to get a good cut so it doesn't get scraggly.

Wardrobes tend to be small. But make sure there is a good range of outfits that are easy to put on and to wear, nothing too tight and uncomfortable, and forget about outfits that have too many fiddly buttons or tight zips that can't be reached. Cosy works well, even for outfits worn inside, especially in the winter (lighter outfits for the summer). Get them scarf, hat, and mittens for outside; a couple of pairs of good shoes; three good nighties; and a comfortable dressing gown that is often worn in public. Ladies like hankies, but they are often lost, so a box of tissues in the room is always a great help.

Also, be aware that it is not a staff responsibility to tidy the drawers but the relatives. Wardrobes need to be gone through regularly and toss out old clothes and shoes and bring new ones in. Staff can get embarrassed having to ask for new clothes, nighties, and underwear, so it is better if you pick up on it first.

Meals and Morning and Afternoon Tea

Relatives are able to stay for meals, but there will generally be a charge that applies. Sometimes staff will let relatives in for a meal without charge, particularly on special occasions. Often, a separate table is set up so you can have some privacy.

One of the first things that often happen when a person goes into a dementia facility is that they put on weight. Morning and afternoon teas are sugary and sweet and the desserts generous and creamy. For many elderly people who are used to eating lightly, it is a shock to the system. Some choose not to eat the fattening food, and their weight stays the same. But many develop a sweet tooth, and eating what is on offer can put on up to five kilograms a month, a staggering amount. If you want to prevent this and the resident does too, then you can request club sandwiches for morning and afternoon tea and fruit for dessert.

Once putting the weight on, it is often hard to lose, so preventing it from being put on in the first place is often the best option. The POA will be asked to fill out meal choices. Include your relative in this process. Options can be considered at that time.

Staff generally offer relatives morning or afternoon tea when they visit, tea or coffee with the accompanying piece of cake or biscuit, even if it is not house policy. They will do so especially if you are a regular visitor and if you arrive right as it is being served.

The Cups

Cups used at morning and afternoon tea vary according to the ability of residents. The main teacup used can often be heavy, poorly designed, and with only an awkward little handle to hold on to. This is difficult to hold for arthritic hands. If the resident is not managing with the smaller cup, progression is made to a much larger cup with a larger handle, but it is often heavy and bulky. The advanced option is a plastic cup.

If your relative is not either managing or liking either option, you can bring in their favourite cup. It may not be an option made publicly but an option nevertheless and a good one. Staff will and do accommodate.

Walking and Going Out

Walks are important, especially for those who are still fit, healthy, and good at walking. They'll want to get outside. For those who aren't, they'll enjoy getting out in a wheelchair.

Managing wheelchairs can be difficult, especially putting them in and out of cars on your own, so having another person like a partner or grandchild with you is always a great help. Even putting walkers in and out of cars can be an effort, especially if you have a bad back.

Another good option is a walk around the grounds. Most places have nice gardens and seats to sit on when you need a rest. The main lounge of the village is always a good place to go and sit and relax. Many have fish ponds or ferneries or some area of interest to enjoy. Some have mini cafes where you can order a coffee and snack food, ideal if getting in and out of the car is difficult.

Power of Attorney Permission

If you don't have time to do it, the POA gives authority to one of the grandchildren to take Grandma out for a walk or an able friend or relative who would also be happy to do it. The grandkids who make the effort to visit, and there are quite a number, would be more than happy to take Granny out in the grounds for a jaunt. If the POA gives permission and the nurse is informed, then all bases are covered.

It is important to give the resident this chance. Able residents get very distressed if they don't get the chance to get outside, and it is the staff that hear their complaints all week, not necessarily the relative when they visit.

Don't Stop Making the Effort

So often, relatives come in regularly at first and then peter out. After a year or two, you see the visits gradually subside, often from the sons, sad to say. Perhaps this is because sons feel awkward or embarrassed with a parent who is 'shut off and shut down', and they don't know what to do. It is unfortunate as they are the ones the residents often spend half their life at the nurses' station calling out for.

Sons like action. If something happens, they will likely join in. Daughters, in contrast, will sit silently and maybe knot or look through a magazine if Mum is not up to much.

Long-Lost Sons

Make it a decent visit when you do come, especially if you haven't visited for ages, not a ten-minute breeze in and breeze out, especially if you haven't seen your mother for ages. Unfortunately, short visits are common, and it leaves the person feeling depressed and disillusioned.

Every mother loves seeing their son (it is mostly the sons they call out for and the daughters who visit), so it is important to make sure it is a good-quality visit. Give them the time to recognise you again, feel your presence, have time to ask you questions (which can often take time to formulate), and 'absorb you' so to speak. Then they can have that reassurance, love, and your presence to keep with them till hopefully the next time.

Supportive Relative Visits

First Group

The longest visits come from the partners living at the same retirement village, often just a short walk away. Many of the husbands spend half the day there as much for themselves as for the wife they are visiting. They are welcomed. They can support their resident wife (though often it is the other way round), have a cup of tea, enjoy the hospitality and the company, and be there when the kids arrive, even if rarely. They often end up enjoying themselves and spending more time at the unit than over at the village. This group often sit in on the morning press readings, join the activities, and sit around watching interesting programmes on the smart TV just like everybody else.

Second Group

This include the working sons and daughters who generally come on the weekends and sometimes after work. Being active, fit, and able, they make the effort to take Mum or Dad out for a walk in the village grounds (wheelchair if needed) or better still out for a car ride and then a walk along the beach or at the park. Ice cream and fish and chips are thrown in if you are lucky. Visit the local cafe and eat out for lunch if the resident is up for it. These are the best visits – outside, in the sun, fresh air. things to see, good company, nice scenery, good food, and something nice to drink. Who doesn't like that?

Other Group

Supportive family, brothers or sisters, and friends (which are often lifelong) are great visitors, often giving respite to the POA and/or main visitor. A range of visits from various people is always the best situation, bringing in new ideas, fresh input, a range of trips out, and lots of enjoyment.

Newspaper

The newspaper is important and highly valued. Only a few lucky residents in the unit get one delivered personally and paid for by the family/trust. Otherwise, only one copy is delivered to the whole unit for use by everyone. It is one of the most important things a POA can do. Keep up the subscription for the newspaper and have it delivered to the village main desk. Labelled with their name on it, staff pick it up daily from there. It is especially important if the person has always been a big reader of it and for the men as they don't have the women's magazines to fall back on.

What Entertainment a Relative Can Provide

Bringing in a friendly little dog is always a thrill, especially the resident's own dog from before they came into the unit. Sharing it around and letting the dog lovers have some time with it is a sure way to get into the good books of everyone.

Well-socialised children are wonderful to have at the unit, especially those who are happy to talk to elderly people. The regular visitors tend to be good at bringing in teenage children but not so much younger children. It is safe for younger children to visit but best if one parent takes them around by hand to visit the residents in the group due to risks of falls. A child taking the dog around for the residents to pat, with parent nearby, is always a double treat.

The interaction and generosity on the part of relatives who befriend the less able and less visited residents, in whatever way, goes a long way to creating a wholesome community. That can be as simple as greeting them by name, smiling and waving, letting them have a pat of the dog, or being happy when they sit at your table when you are having a chat and a cup of tea with their family member.

Zoom

If going overseas, Zoom is popular especially since Covid-19. You really need another employed carer to be there for these calls as the staff don't have enough time to be there for the whole call, unless it is short. Staff can set up the call on the unit's laptop device, but for the call itself, it is best if someone else is there in support.

If overseas and you are employing outside carers, you can talk to them on the Zoom call and get updated. This way, you can keep your finger on the pulse. Seeing your parent, you can observe if they need a haircut. Have they lost weight? How is their mood? A lot of bases can be covered with a Zoom call.

Workshops

Some visiting relatives attend morning newspaper readings and what the residents call 'thinking workshops', but others choose not to. It is personal preference as long as the resident is getting a quality visit and not being taken away from an engaging activity just to be sat by an uncommunicative relative spending all the time on their iPhone (does happen).

Meeting and Greeting

Don't come up and slap your mother on both shoulders from behind and say, 'Mum, I'm here!' Maybe it's all right at home, where she is not likely to see anyone else for the rest of the day, but not in a busy unit. It could be anyone, including residents ready to assault.

Also, don't expect her to recognise you from a 'hi, Mum'. There's plenty of 'hi, Mums' going on all around, so don't expect yours to necessarily stand out.

Be mindful that they may have forgotten your name, especially if you haven't been in for a while. So the best way is to come up to them and greet them face to face so they can actually see you. Come forward from their front, lean down so they can actually see you, and say, 'Hi, Mum. It's Matt. Great to see you.' Give your name. It saves them from embarrassment if they've forgotten or can't recall it at that moment.

Then all bases are covered. They can see that it is indeed you. Of course, how could they possibly forget? And they have the name right there too. 'Matt, it is so good to see you, darling.'

Farewells

Saying goodbye is emotional for many. It can upset them for days if it is a bad one. The best farewell is after a good-quality visit. Say, you've been at the unit for an hour; then it is a good idea to say ten minutes before you go that you will be going soon. That gives your mother time to psychologically prepare and also time enough to ask anything she might have been wanting to ask before you leave or even for you to direct her to the toilet before you go, which is always helpful. It saves them from having to find someone else yet again to guide them.

Let them come to the door with you to say goodbye. Don't just sneak off and think they don't notice. Better still and a favourite for the regular visitors is getting a window seat for them overlooking the car park just before they go. Then assuming the resident can see the car park from the window, they can wave to you from the window before you get in the car to take off. Everyone loves that.

If not, then ensure that you get them to a good seat somewhere else before you leave. The best seat is by one of their friends, whom you will, by now, be recognising, so they can beam in pride to tell them that, yes, you arrived as they have been saying all along that they would. Don't just leave them sitting in the corner of an empty room on leaving. Set them up for the next step.

Assess the needs and use your common sense. You know your relative better than anyone. Work with the staff but still hold true to what you know is important for your relative and their needs. Exchanging knowledge and information is the growing strength of any community and not least at a dementia unit, where relatives and friends are a big part of that.

Biographical Note

Physiotherapy gives a particular spatial and practical intelligence for understanding how best to help someone with dementia. Having a physiotherapy business for twenty-five years treating muscle- and mental-tension-related OOS (occupational overuse syndrome) / RSI (repetitive strain injury) gave me a head start in understanding stress, so once understanding the stress aspect of dementia, I had the confidence to deal with it.

Physiotherapists are problem-solvers, enabling patients to self-manage through effort and hard work. This ethos I've applied to the dementia community, which can flourish on the basis of their improved individual concentration and confidence, as well as better communication and consideration for one another, enabling them to create their own unique and caring community. For all these reasons, the residents' efforts deserve credit for explaining their dementia experience to me and being prepared to work hard to improve their capacity and capability as individuals and as a community.

www.pietavalentine.com

Acknowledgements

My immense thanks firstly goes to my committed and loving parents.

My mother Adair Valentine (a former nurse) encouraged me to be a physiotherapist and my scholarly father Dr John Valentine was a liberal GP who supported every twist and turn of my multifarious ventures.

From him I developed my love of reading and life long learning.

Throughout my physiotherapy years I have had many tutors, teachers and employers (too vast to mention) who have helped me develop the art of observation and assessment, essential where no medication and only physical and psychological modalities are used.

With the thousands of patients I have treated over thirty five years, more than ten of those years was spent working with geriatrics, many of whom had dementia.

This work has provided ample material for both books and their detailed epilogues.

Travel to many far flung places, and living on four different continents over the past four decades has given me the ability to have a range of insights, I wouldn't have otherwise had.

Enormous thanks to the late Stephen Stratford who edited The Residents' Voice with empathy and insight, with his colleague Paul Litterick completing the edit.

The library staff at Sumner and Linwood libraries have assisted tirelessly with book research, technology and timely advice.

Trish Summerfield has excelled as a reader and helped me see the importance of keeping the dementia residents' voice and rise, central to the novels and epilogues.

Since in Christchurch my supportive friend the late lawyer Rob Davidson introduced me to criminal lawyer Peter Doody who educated me with his sharp eye and attention to detail in regards to the novels.

GP Dr Kathy Davey a friend and a toast master colleague for many years has provided intelligent dialogue around the multifarious issues of dementia.

And to all the others who have helped throughout the years, too many to mention. Thank you.